A CONSUMER'S GUIDE TO **MEMS** & **NANO**TECHNOLOGY

MARLENE BOURNE

Bourne Research LLC
Scottsdale, AZ

Cover by Nocturnal Graphic Design

ISBN-10: 0-9795505-4-8
ISBN-13: 978-0-9795505-4-6

Library of Congress Control Number: 2007902860

Published by Bourne Research LLC
8867 E. Mountain Spring Rd, Scottsdale, AZ 85255
www.bourneresearch.com

Printed in the United States of America

August 2007

First Edition

10 9 8 7 6 5 4 3 2 1

To Lou Naturman

For starting me on this fantastic voyage

CONTENTS

PART II
COOL PRODUCTS AVAILABLE TODAY

11 • HEALTHCARE   215

ACKNOWLEDGEMENTS

My sincerest thanks to:

Jessica Dixon and Howard Lovy for their editing assistance,

All of the professors, researchers and companies for kindly allowing me to include their images in this book,

My friends and co-workers, for cheerfully enduring my endless talk about MEMS and nanotechnology,

And especially, "the mom."

PREFACE

Welcome to the wonderful world of really small stuff. Things so tiny, that it takes special microscopes to even see them. I became involved with MEMS (MicroElectroMechanical Systems) and nanotechnology quite by accident more than a decade ago, and it's been my passion ever since. This is partly because I talk with companies every day about products they're developing that are so cutting edge, in many cases, they won't be on the market for at least another ten years; maybe more.

So, what is nanotechnology? What are MEMS? And how are they changing the way we live, work and play?

In Part 1 of this book, I take you into the micro-world (and beyond) to look at an amazing range of unimaginably small sensors, structures, materials and more that scientists and engineers around the world have spent decades developing. In doing so, I will address the fundamental questions of: What exactly are they? How do they work? Why is smaller better? And who's developing all of these cool things?

Part 2 provides an in-depth look at where MEMS and nanotechnology are already found, and the difference they're making in all sorts of products. From cars and TVs, to sporting goods and even wheelchairs, MEMS and nanotechnology are enabling the creation of products that are smaller, smarter, lighter, stronger and more unique than ever before.

This isn't the stuff of science fiction, and I'm not talking about the fantastical products of tomorrow; rather, the examples I provide are real items available for purchase today.

Over the course of my career, I've developed an enormous respect for the scientists and engineers who create all of these incredible things. What they're doing, and the products we can buy as a result, is unbelievably cool.

I'm certain you'll think so too.

PART 1

AN OVERVIEW OF MEMS
AND NANOTECHNOLOGY

We predict the future. And the best way to predict the future is to invent it.

—*Well-Manicured Man (The X-Files, 1995)*

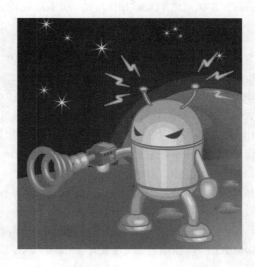

1 • AN INTRODUCTION TO NANO/MEMS

The results of my high school career test shocked me. Right at the top of the list was engineering. Are you kidding me? An *engineer*? I wanted to be a fashion designer. Fast forward twenty years, and it seems that test was right. I never did pursue engineering, but I might as well have. Today, I'm immersed in it.

For more than a decade now, I've been following the latest developments in chemical, electrical and mechanical engineering as they move from the research lab into real products. And a lot of these things are now finding their way into clothes. Go figure.

It's easy for me to say that MEMS (MicroElectroMechanical Systems) and nanotechnology are truly changing how we live, work and play; but what does that really mean?

Are you curious why sunscreen, which used to be white, is now clear? How motion-sensing cell phones work? Why your car knows when to deploy the airbags? How liquids bead up and roll off some surfaces? Why silver nanoparticles are such a big deal?

The answers to those questions (and a whole lot more), come courtesy of two emerging areas of engineering and science: MEMS and nanotechnology. Unfortunately, from my perspective, what many people read about MEMS and nanotechnology, and what they actually understand, are two entirely different things. This is because most of the stories I see in the press focus on the gee-whiz "what ifs" and "imagine this" angles.

But, let's take a step back and see how today's next-generation technologies are going to get us to that fantastic future.

I wrote this book to peek behind the mysterious curtain surrounding the science. In doing so, I felt a little like Dorothy when she looked behind the curtain and found the Wizard of Oz. The special effects of Oz were cool, but there's something even more interesting about how they really work—even if it's just a man pulling levers and pushing buttons. Taking the time to discuss what MEMS and nanotechnology are, in a non-scientific way, will not only give you a greater understanding of their use, but the benefits that they offer; both today *and* for the future.

The bottom line is that these components, materials and processes are making products smaller, smarter, lighter, stronger and more unique than ever before. You will get a detailed look at not only the where and how, but more importantly, *why* these technologies are being used.

Since bursting onto the scene a few years ago (at least according to articles in the popular press), nanotechnology has quickly become an umbrella term for everything small. As a result, two entirely separate disciplines, one comprising science and the other engineering, now fall under the nanotechnology spectrum. A lot of what is referred to as "nanotech" is actually the result of a completely different technology: MEMS.

Why bother to distinguish between the two? Does the difference really even matter?

For the general public, especially those who are curious about how things work, you'll find the difference interesting, but it won't *matter*. The distinction is important for those within the business and financial communities, because MEMS are playing an increasingly important role in the commercialization of nanotechnology; in some instances, one is not possible without the other.

One of the best examples of this convergence is the atomic force microscope, which allows us to create images at the nanoscale, and is driving the understanding and production of nanoscale materials and structures. But the tiny tips that create those images are MEMS devices.

Perhaps most telling is what is taking place at the research level. More universities (such as Albany Nanotech, UC Berkeley, Cornell University, and Georgia Tech, to name just a few) are now conducting research in both areas, concurrently, within the same facility. So, to appreciate the full scope of nanotechnology, one must ultimately understand MEMS as well.

What Are MEMS?

MicroElectroMechanical Systems. That's quite a tongue twister; yet it's fairly straightforward. MEMS are basically micrometer-sized structures which combine both a mechanical component and electronic circuitry on a single chip. MEMS' origins are well-rooted within the semiconductor industry, so the fabrication processes are basically the same as those used to create integrated circuits (ICs).

But what makes them different—what can MEMS do that semiconductors can't? For the most part, semiconductors (such as microprocessors and microcontrollers) are the brains behind electronic products. But MEMS are the eyes, ears, arms and legs that help the brain know what is going on and decide what to do.

There are a number of different ways to fabricate MEMS, but the three primary methods are surface micromachining, bulk micromachining and deep reactive ion etching (DRIE). The biggest difference between these processes and those for semi-conductors is basically that the processing steps (the etches) are deeper. This is because, unlike an IC, which is two-dimensional, MEMS are three-dimensional; in effect, you're essentially "sculpting" a silicon wafer.

With surface micromachining, thin films deposited on a silicon wafer are selectively etched to create the structures desired. Layers of material (masks) are deposited or "grown" on top of one another, each of which has a different pattern. Parts of the masks (or even entire layers) are then etched away by either photolithography, acid, ionized gas or plasma. Simple designs need only a few masks, but more complicated ones can use up to 100. The end result is that the MEMS device is basically built *on top* of the wafer.

Bulk micromachining is completely different because the silicon wafer itself is etched away to create the structure. The etching process is the same, but the end result is that the MEMS device is created *inside* the wafer.

Deep reactive ion etching is an extension of bulk micro-machining, but the difference is the creation of MEMS devices with very high aspect ratios, generally 20:1 or more.

While most MEMS devices today are silicon, other materials are used too, including plastic, glass, ceramic and metal. Some of the more novel materials I've seen include silicone (rubber) and even diamond. But what gives MEMS its cost advantage is the ability to mass produce these devices via silicon wafers, just like semi-conductors; and in many instances, using the same equipment.

As with semiconductors, the dimensions of MEMS devices are microscale, falling squarely within the range of 1 to 100 microns, which is generally smaller than a human hair. In most cases, the entire MEMS device falls within this size range, although I've come across examples in which the overall structure may exceed 100 microns, with only certain aspects of it being microscale, but those are generally exceptions.

Most MEMS devices also have moving parts, but some have none. The majority of those that have no moving parts typically deal with the movement of fluid. So, the design of MEMS themselves can range from something as simple as a channel (which obviously doesn't move) to unbelievably complex, intricate structures (which you'll see later) that do.

Despite the "electro" piece of the acronym, which implies the use of electricity, a few MEMS devices are actually powered by magnetics. This is fairly rare, but it's important to point out that the power source doesn't determine whether or not it's a MEMS device; from my point of view, it's primarily all about the fabrication method or process.

The materials used, whether there are moving parts or not and the source of power is all insignificant; what's key about MEMS devices is that they perform a mechanical function. Some move fluid, others move light, still others sense vibration or pressure. The diversity of MEMS devices created to date is nothing short of amazing, ranging from nozzles (basically holes) to intricate locking mechanisms that prevent nuclear warheads from accidentally going off.

What is Nanotechnology?

There are all sorts of definitions for nanotechnology, ranging from "the manipulation of atoms and molecules" to "the ability to measure, see, manipulate and manufacture things between 1 and 100 nanometers." At its core, nanotechnology is all about materials; more specifically, leveraging the unique properties a material has at the nanoscale.

And how small, exactly, is that? Most sources specify that any material or structure with dimensions of 1 to 100 nanometers is considered nanotechnology.

That's pretty straightforward, right? Not so fast. I've found that much of what's labeled nanotech technically isn't. A far broader definition of nanotechnology is generally being applied: basically, *anything* whose physical dimensions are measured in nanometers. The end result is that both micro and nano are frequently used to describe the same thing.

How is this possible? Well, it's easier than you might think. Let's take a particle with a diameter of 300 nanometers. I've found such particles commonly referred to as both a microparticle and as a nanoparticle. Technically, both are correct.

There's a fuzzy area that connects the micro and nano worlds: sub-micron. One can refer to the above example as a microparticle, because it has a diameter of 0.3 microns. It can also be referred to as a nanoparticle, because an alternative way to state its size is 300 nanometers. So, while this particle isn't technically nanotechnology per the myriad of definitions out there, it's certainly nano*scale*. There seems to be an assumption that anything measurable in nanometers falls within the scope of nanotechnology.

This is a very important distinction due to growing concerns about the use of nanotechnology in consumer products, and cosmetics in particular. As you will see, many of the ingredients in use are measured in nanometers, but they're technically sub-micron. So, that raises the question: is it appropriate to label all matter with nanoscale dimensions nanotechnology?

Not according to ASTM International, whose published standard defines nanoscale as having dimensions of 1 to 100 nanometers[1]. But just because a technical standards body creates a definition, it doesn't mean that manufacturers or even the general public, will follow suit. Using the term nanometer, even to describe a sub-micron particle, will likely result in that particle being viewed as nanotechnology, regardless of whether industry deems it to be nano or not.

What makes this matter even more confusing is the frequent description of nanotechnology as the manipulation of atoms and molecules. While this is correct to a certain extent, what we're really talking about in this case is the general concept of nanoscience; the study of things at the nanoscale. This not only includes nanotechnology, but basic biology and chemistry as well.

The bottom line is this: nanoscale is simply a form of measurement, which ranges from 1 to 999 nanometers. Nanotechnology is the ability to precisely produce or manufacture materials and structures with dimensions of 1 to 100 nanometers, in order to leverage the unique properties they exhibit at that size.

Let's take a journey into the micro- and nano-world to see what I'm talking about. The following seven images really put MEMS and nanotechnology into perspective by looking at what we might find on the head of a straight pin (which is about 1–2 millimeters in diameter), by magnifying it one million times its original size.

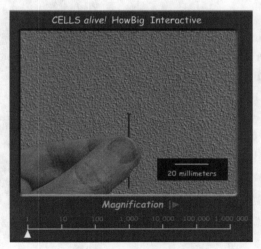

Image courtesy of Quill Graphics

If we magnify the pin by a factor of 10, we not only see a human hair (the diameter of which ranges in size from roughly 60 to 120 microns), but we can just make out a tiny spec; this is a dust mite, whose width is about 200 microns (also called micrometers).

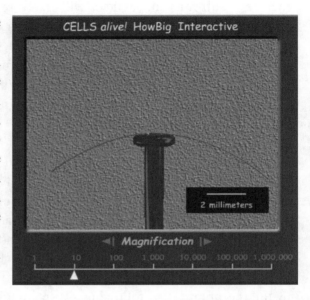

Zooming in by another factor of 10, or now 100 times the original size, the scale of the dust mite and hair are much more apparent. The tiny speck in the middle is a grain of pollen.

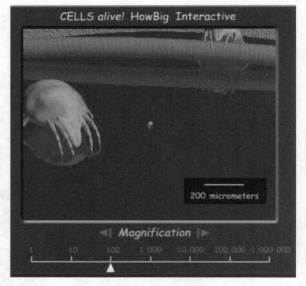

Images courtesy of Quill Graphics

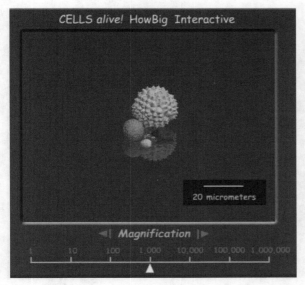

By magnifying the pin 1,000 times, we now see the pollen grain towers over several other items: a white blood cell (left), a grain of brewer's yeast, and a red blood cell (right).

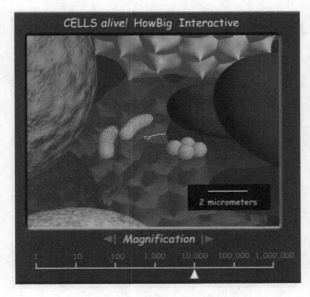

Magnifying our pin once again, we see that the red blood cell (right) dwarfs two objects which turn out to be bacteria: the two caterpillar-shaped items are E. coli, and the 4 balls are staphylococcus. But, what's that string-like object?

Images courtesy of Quill Graphics

The head of our pin is now magnified 100,000 times its original size. The string-like object we see is a virus—the Ebola virus to be exact. And the four tiny balls next to it? Those are the rhinovirus, the nasty little bug behind the common cold.

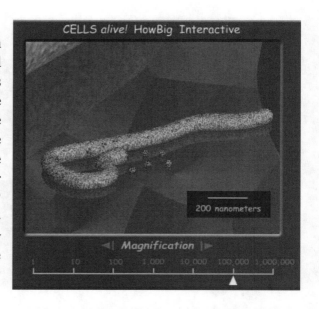

Magnifying our pin one last time, we see how small the cold virus really is. Keep in mind that the scale of this last image is one million times smaller than the one we started out with. Here is where we could see buckyballs or carbon nanotubes, which are just a few nanometers in diameter.

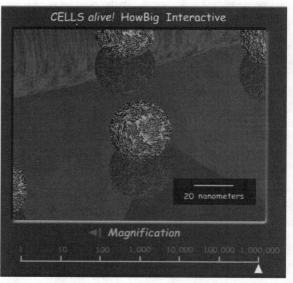

Images courtesy of Quill Graphics

These images help to illustrate that while things like viruses and bacteria are indeed nanoscale, they aren't nanotechnology. Only things that are purposefully manufactured at this scale are.

You might also recognize that while nanotechnology is indeed really small, so are things at the microscale. So it makes sense then that you'd ask: how much difference is there really between a microparticle and a nanoparticle? What's the big deal?

Let me put this into perspective in another way, using an example that helped me to understand it better: elephants and mice. For illustrative purposes, let's pretend that a particle 10 microns in diameter is the size of an elephant, and that a particle 10 nanometers in diameter is the size of a mouse. Already you can see that there is a tremendous size difference; just as you saw the size difference between a red blood cell and a virus.

As you move from the micro- to the nano-world, the physical, chemical and biological properties of a material changes. How they work and the properties they exhibit as a microparticle, are very different from how they work and the properties they exhibit as a nanoparticle.

Take gold for example. At the microscale, it absorbs red and blue light, and looks yellow. With a diameter of just 30 nanometers, it absorbs blue and yellow light, and looks red. Another good example is zinc oxide, which is commonly used as a sunscreen. As a microparticle, it's an opaque white; as a nanoparticle, it's transparent. Because it's now clear, it can be added to all sorts of products without changing how they look; which is why it is more widely used in cosmetics.

One of the most important properties of a nanoscale material is surface area. So, if you have a one-ton microparticle (the elephant), versus one ton of nanoparticles (the mice), you have far more surface area for the same amount of weight. Here's a good example of this. Let's say you have two sugar cubes. Now, crush one.

The big sugar cube is like the elephant. All of the little crystals from the crushed sugar cube are like the mice. You have an equal amount of sugar, but the crushed sugar has more surface area.

This is how the use of "nano" results in materials that are stronger, lighter, thinner, more transparent, etc. And you will use a lot less of that material. In addition, you can do things with the nanoparticles that you couldn't with the microparticle—like coating or encapsulating other materials.

What about nanobots, nanoelectronics and nanosensors? Well, with the exception of nanobots, a medical application I'll address later, the other two actually fit into a third category: NEMS.

NEMS (NanoElectroMechanical Systems) are the convergence of MEMS and nanotechnology. In other words, it's a product in which a MEMS device and nanomaterials (or nanostructures) are key components. The bottom line is that you need both.

Many sensors, especially those that sense biological and chemical compounds, now fall into this category, as do two products that are very successful commercially: the atomic force microscope and a cool device called lab-on-a-chip.

A Brief History

Since the roots of MEMS are squarely planted within the semiconductor industry, its foundation is traceable to 1947, with the invention of the transistor at Bell Labs. A transistor, which controls electrical current, is the basic building block of today's electronic products; we wouldn't have them otherwise.

In 1954, the discovery of the piezoresistive effect (the change in a material's resistance in response to stress) in silicon and germanium by Dr. Charles S. Smith[2] really laid the cornerstone for MEMS sensor development. This led to the creation of silicon strain gauges (a sensor that measures force), which two companies, Kulite and Honeywell, began selling in 1958.

The following year, in 1959, physicist Richard Feynman gave his now legendary speech where he talked about the possibility of one day working with tools and processes at the molecular level[3].

Throughout the 1960s, considerable research pertaining to MEMS fabrication took place (even though the acronym had not yet been coined). During the 1965–1967 timeframe, the concept of micromachining was born, although the term didn't formally come into play until around 1982. First, in 1965, came the demonstrated use of a sacrificial layer, the precursor to surface micromachining. Two years later, in 1967, came anisotropic etching, part of the technique that's now called bulk micromachining. Kulite and Honeywell used both techniques in the late 1960s and early 1970s to fabricate their strain gauges.

Two significant events occurred in 1974: National Semiconductor began selling the first silicon pressure sensor (still not called MEMS), and Norio Taniguchi, a professor at Tokyo Science University, coined the term "nanotechnology" when predicting the use of micromachining in the formation of structures smaller than 100 nanometers[4].

During the 1980s several breakthroughs took place which opened the door to nanotechnology research. In 1980 came the invention of the scanning tunneling microscope, an instrument that allowed scientists to see atomic structures *and* maneuver them. Shortly thereafter, in 1985, Harry Kroto and Richard Smalley discovered the buckyball. In 1986 came the invention of a second tool that's become critical to the understanding (and commercialization) of nanotechnology: the atomic force microscope. This instrument measures the topography (or hills and valleys) of a surface via an extremely tiny probe or pointed tip.

The term MEMS finally made its first appearance at a conference in July 1987, although no one is specifically credited with the creation of the acronym (or the long version). However, its use is not universal; the Japanese actually use the term "micromachines" (amongst several others), whereas Europeans prefer "micro-systems." It's important to note that the term microsystems often includes products that are not produced via MEMS fabrication techniques; as such, it's a much broader term that encompasses more than just MEMS.

In 1991, two more events took place that really got things rolling for both the MEMS and nanotechnology industries: discovery of the carbon nanotube (or at least generating wider awareness of them) by NEC researcher Sumio Iijima and the commercial launch of MEMS accelerometers.

Hype, Part I (aka The Bug Years)

The early 1990s were initially a time of considerable excitement for MEMS, but it turned sour fairly quickly, resulting in the entire industry basically going underground. By the time I began writing my first market report on the technology, in the mid 1990s, the industry was starting to emerge from this "dark" period. So, what exactly happened?

From what I can tell, MEMS experienced its first round of real hype around 1990–1991 as the media caught on to this amazing technology that allowed for the fabrication of microscale devices. While gathering information at the time, what I recall most vividly is that nearly every story I came across in the press tied this wondrous technological approach to the 1966 classic film "Fantastic Voyage". The movie, starring Raquel Welch, is about how a team of scientists in a submarine are shrunk down to microscopic size and injected into the body of a dying man in order to save his life.

The concept of MEMS, and its possibilities, resulted in the notion that in the not-too-distant future, microbots would soon be running rampant through our bodies, fighting disease in a way that was the stuff of science fiction. It truly was "fantastic."

Photographs showing dust mites and ants towering over MEMS devices to demonstrate their extremely small scale only served to highlight this. But MEMS devices were still at the very earliest stages of commercialization, and simply couldn't live up to the enormous hype and expectations that came about as a result.

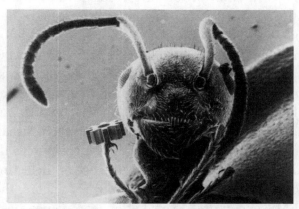

Ant with MEMS gear. © *Copyright 2007 Forschungszentrum Karlsruhe.*

For all intents and purposes, the industry simply stopped talking. In fact, there was clearly a period of time in which there was virtually no press at all. Keep in mind that, in the early 1990s, few venture capitalists were funding MEMS start-ups, and public relations efforts were virtually non-existent. What happened is that companies hunkered down and focused on product development; with unprecedented support from the U.S. government.

The Defense Advanced Research Projects Agency (DARPA), formed in 1958, is tasked with identifying emerging, innovative, revolutionary technologies critical to U.S. national security. By the early 1990s, MEMS was identified as such a technology.

In 1992, DARPA launched a program focused on applying MEMS to various military platforms and tapped Dr. Kaigham (Ken) Gabriel, a professor at Carnegie Mellon University, to head the effort. During his five-year tenure, its annual budget grew to more than $70 million. Because so many companies (primarily start-ups) received grants from DARPA in those days, I've frequently referred to DARPA as the original venture capitalist of the MEMS industry.

It was a win-win for all involved. MEMS start-ups used DARPA's program as a way to fund early product development efforts, and the military benefited from the application of next-generation technologies (such as the gyro sensor, which was developed for use in smart bombs). After the project was complete, the start-up basically had a finished product ready for sale.

By the late-1990s, commercialization was on a roll and MEMS were going mainstream. The years of concerted research efforts were paying off as more devices made their way into the market, and more markets began to embrace the use of these tiny pressure sensors, accelerometers, lab-on-a-chip, gyro sensors, thermopiles, optical MEMS and more. Even better, companies began talking about their product development again.

With increased visibility in the press, more companies made a concerted effort to move beyond the bug photos, which by then had become synonymous with MEMS. The industry was clearly growing up. But shaking the "bug-on-a-chip" science project moniker proved difficult. Some embraced the bugs, others railed against them. In terms of research, it was a great way to make engineering cool; but from a business perspective, it was an increasingly sensitive issue.

With venture capitalists starting to look more seriously at MEMS as an investment opportunity, and the fact that the technology was rapidly gaining respect as a bona fide disruptor to an increasing number of markets, image was a concern. The tide seemed to turn when Forbes ASAP devoted almost an entire issue to MEMS, culminating in a photo of a MEMS device on the cover of the April 2, 2001 issue. MEMS had indeed arrived.

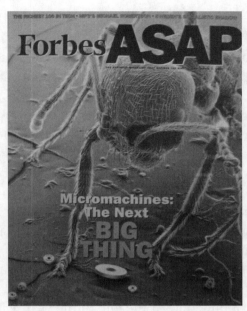

Reprinted by Permission of FORBES ASAP Magazine
© 2007 Forbes Media LLC

Unfortunately, to the dismay of some, its poster child was a "damn ant." Personally, I was a little torn. I was thrilled to see that MEMS was the cover story, but part of me kind of wished another image had been used. Yet, there are few that tell the story so well. The bug photos generate an immediate "that's cool" factor. Most people know how big an ant is, so such photos provide a great perspective of how small MEMS really are.

Hype, Part II (aka VCs Gone Wild)

At the time the Forbes ASAP issue hit the newsstands, the MEMS industry was reaching the zenith of a second round of hype. But this time, things were different. A decade earlier, the hype was all about the possibilities. This second round of hype was all about real products.

In 1998, venture capital (VC) firms provided MEMS start-ups with roughly $100 million; just two years later, that number exploded to more than $1.2 billion. Of course, much of this was due to the anticipated boom taking place in optical networking—an application in which optical MEMS (tiny mirrors) were going to play a pivotal role.

That same year, 2000, saw some of the richest MEMS acquisitions ever. Nortel Networks acquired Xros for $3.25 billion in March, followed a month later with the acquisition of Cronos Integrated Microsystems by JDS Uniphase for $750 million. A few weeks after that, Corning acquired Intellisense for $500 million. Not so coincidentally, all three were developing MEMS devices for use in optical networking.

By early 2001, even as the MEMS industry was enjoying its status as a bona fide technology that would change the world, the bottom was dropping out. At the end of the year, with the telecom crash, MEMS became a four-letter word; and not in a good sense.

The only reason for this really was MEMS' close affiliation with telecommunications. The excitement about next-generation optical networks quickly generated a level of hype and expectation that couldn't be met. As a component that could help make that a reality, MEMS were swept up in the tide. This was the next big thing. I look back at the telecom forecasts from that time (including mine), and can only shake my head.

What ultimately happened is that MEMS became too closely identified with the bursting of another tech bubble, and the damage was done. VC funding dropped dramatically, reaching just $100 million in 2003. This occurred concurrently with an unprecedented level of consolidation. More than four dozen MEMS start-ups went dark during this period, although most of them were almost exclusively focused on optical networking, including new fabrication facilities hoping for a piece of the action.

However, despite the company closures, a notable number of start-ups actually entered the MEMS industry during this period as well, but getting VC interest (much less any money) was tough, to say the least. While the MEMS industry struggled with another round of bad press and its lowest VC funding in five years, nanotechnology funding actually reached an all-time high, at a little more than $300 million.

Perhaps not so coincidentally, at the same time, media interest in nanotechnology soared. The press caught whiff of an emerging technology that, like MEMS, had the potential to be incredibly disruptive. Stories began to proliferate about this thing called nanotechnology, and it seemed like every story talked about how *nanobots* would soon be used to fight disease in our bodies, just like that 1966 movie, "Fantastic Voyage."

Sound familiar?

From my perspective, it was déja-vu all over again. But more interestingly, MEMS somehow became mixed up with nanotechnology. I think this confusion took place when reports of IBM's Millipede project started to hit the press. While it was clear in this case that MEMS *enabled* nanotechnology, somehow the distinction became fuzzy, and MEMS suddenly became a *type* of nanotechnology. It's the classic telephone game in play—you start out with a message, and when passed along, it changes.

Either way, I found myself fielding more calls to talk about the MEMS segment of nanotechnology. In my opinion, it was especially important to keep the two separated because the research, development, production, integration, time-to-market, supply chain, and overall cost involved, was—and still is—completely different. These factors should be important to those within the financial community, both VCs and investors alike.

A Period of Transition

By late 2003, nanotechnology reached the zenith of its first real round of hype. In fact, its parallels with the hype MEMS experienced in the early 1990s were almost eerie, to the point where funding of nanotech start-ups dropped just a year later as VCs quickly realized that the hype didn't live up to the expectations generated. That is, the commercialization of nanotechnology was further out than initially thought.

The biggest difference for nanotechnology start-ups was that VCs and public relations firms were on board almost from the very beginning, a far cry from MEMS' early days. As such, nanotech companies seemed to weather the hype storm a little bit better.

What's been most interesting to watch is the 180-degree turn in press coverage pertaining to nanotechnology, and in a relatively short period of time. By late 2005, whispers began to emerge about environmental impacts and safety concerns. In just two years, nanotechnology went from being heralded as one of the most wondrous scientific breakthroughs in modern times, to being referred to as the next asbestos. Not exactly a good thing.

As for MEMS, 2004 and 2005 were banner years for the industry. During this time, 29 companies were acquired for more than $2 billion, with acquisition activity basically split evenly over the two-year period. It was, in a word, unprecedented; but not entirely unexpected.

MEMS start-ups have not only been viewed as external research labs for larger companies, but they also compete directly with them. (This is quite different from nanotech start-ups, who are generally suppliers to big firms.) So, there's a long history of acquisitions in the MEMS industry. In fact, only a handful of MEMS start-ups have ever gone public.

Where We Are Now

Commercially speaking, nanotechnology really is in its earliest stages; at the same time, its use is far more ubiquitous than many realize. To a certain extent, despite being more mature, the same holds true for MEMS. Although the integration of both is quite broad, their use isn't terribly deep. That is, only a few models in any particular product category actually benefit from nano-materials and/or MEMS at this time. But this isn't surprising.

The adoption curve basically mandates that companies will leverage new materials and/or processes in just a handful of products first—these are typically luxury items for early adopters. The length of time for new approaches to be adapted for mass products for the general public takes time. And the more cost-sensitive the product (i.e. consumer electronics), the greater amount of time it will take before products for the average consumer will benefit from and/or use these new technologies.

As you're about to see, we're almost there.

The nice thing about standards is that there are so many of them to choose from.

—Andrew S. Tanenbaum

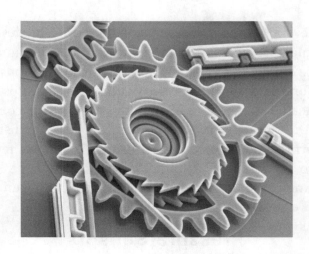

2 • MEMS
(MICROELECTROMECHANICAL SYSTEMS)

After nearly three decades in the making, it's hard to believe that MEMS devices are not yet considered mainstream—close, but not quite. Despite having found extensive use in the automotive, computing and industrial segments, two key markets remain virtually untapped: consumer electronics and medicine. But the MEMS industry is tantalizingly close to conquering those markets as well. MEMS devices are slowly finding their way into products like cell phones, TVs, asthma inhalers and wheelchairs.

Engineers have long applied various micromachining techniques to create, develop and produce an amazingly diverse array of MEMS devices. Some are incredibly simple, whereas others are unbelievably complex. The most common are pressure and inertial sensors, as well as ink jet printer heads, which combined make up the bulk of MEMS sales—more than $7.8 billion in 2006. But, this is just the tip of the iceberg.

With several hundred companies involved in the development and manufacture of MEMS devices worldwide, the industry is a classic case of David vs. Goliath. Large, multinational firms currently account for the majority of sales, but small start-ups often go head-to-head with them, and in some cases, with considerable success. Due to the competitive nature of the industry, these smaller firms tend to be acquired, which is why so few MEMS start-ups or "pure-plays" are publicly traded.

Let's explore the "micro" devices of this fascinating micro-world a little more closely.

Pressure Sensors

Pressure sensors are pretty straightforward—they measure the pressure of gas, liquid, vapor and even dust. This is generally done by monitoring how much an extremely thin membrane moves while under pressure. If there's no pressure, it doesn't move at all. Under high pressure, it will bend significantly.

Take a tissue and place it tightly over the top of a glass. Now, lightly place your finger on it. Do you see it move? That's a little bit like the motion a membrane experiences in the presence of low pressure. The more pressure you apply, the more the tissue bends. This is what occurs under high pressure.

MEMS pressure sensors are able to detect anything from no pressure at all to pressures of more than 60,000 pounds per square inch (psi). Low pressure sensing most frequently comes into play in automated heating, cooling and ventilation (HVAC) systems to monitor airflow; such as the air that comes out of the vent when your heater or air conditioner is on. High pressure applications are generally industrial in nature, like the water jets used in food processing. This is similar to the spray head you might have on your garden hose, or when you place your thumb over the hose to make the water spray harder.

MEMS pressure sensors got their start back in 1974 when National Semiconductor began selling them to automotive manufacturers for the monitoring of Manifold Absolute Pressure (MAP) in car engines. By 1982, they were finding their way into another high volume application: disposable blood pressure sensing. It's costly to sterilize and re-use medical equipment, and doctors need to monitor the blood pressure of patients during surgical procedures. So the medical community quickly embraced this particular application.

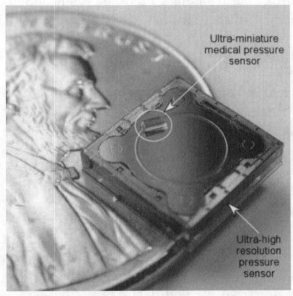

Two MEMS pressure sensors. Photo courtesy of Integrated Sensing Systems, Inc.

Today, MEMS pressure sensors derive the bulk of their revenue from use in automotive and industrial applications; however, due to their small size, they're also found in products as varied as cell phones, watches and scuba equipment, as well as all sorts of medical instruments and other unique medical devices.

Several dozen companies worldwide manufacture MEMS pressure sensors, with most focused on a specific market. For example, the really expensive pressure sensors used in industrial manufacturing are sold by companies such as Emerson Electric, GE Sensing, Schneider Electric and Yokogawa. On the other hand, Robert Bosch, Freescale Semiconductor and Infineon Technologies supply pressure sensors for use in automotive applications.

The companies who manufacture pressure sensors for use in medical and consumer applications tend to be more specialized, and range from big firms like Freescale Semiconductor and GE Sensing, to smaller specialty firms like Measurement Specialties and Silicon Microstructures.

Inertial Sensors

Inertial sensors measure inertia—which is another word for movement. This can range from subtle, like the vibration generated by a running motor, to the obvious, such as the swing of your arm; or even the shock generated if you were to walk into a wall. The two types of MEMS sensors that detect inertia are accelerometers and gyroscopes (which are simply referred to as gyros).

Accelerometers

An accelerometer measures linear or two-dimensional movement along one of three axes: X, Y and Z. Consider a sliding glass door: it can move left or right, just like the X axis. If you take a step forward or backward through the door, that's the Y axis. If you bend your knees into a squat and then strand up straight, that up and down movement is the Z axis. These sensors can also measure tilt. When you open the door of an oven, it tilts outward; both the X and Z axis can measure that angle.

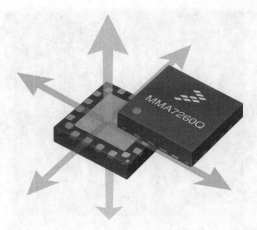

Two-dimensional accelerometer movement. Photo courtesy Freescale Semiconductor.

While the sensing itself is fairly straightforward, from a design standpoint, these sensors are pretty complex. Most look like two interlocked hair combs, which may be one reason why they're referred to as comb drives. Considering that the dimensions of each of these structures within the overall sensor are just a few micrometers wide, the ability to manufacture these devices is that much more incredible.

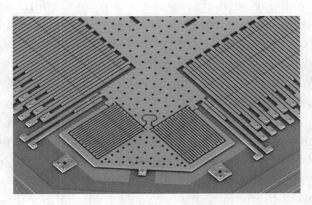

Top view of an accelerometer. Copyright Analog Devices, Inc. All rights reserved.

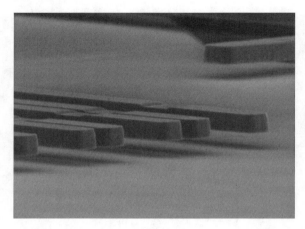

Accelerometer "fingers." Copyright Analog Devices, Inc. All rights reserved.

Accelerometers got their start in 1970, when Kulite first demonstrated the technology, but they weren't commercialized until 1991, when Analog Devices began selling them as the trigger mechanism in the airbags of passenger cars. A few years later, in 1996, gyros made their debut in high-end luxury cars as a way to provide stability during tight cornering and on slippery roads.

A new generation of accelerometers is now emerging; so despite being around for several decades, innovation continues to take place. Accelerometers available today can measure one, two or all three axes. Dual-axis accelerometers are by far the most common, and are available from several dozen companies. Leading suppliers include Analog Devices, Robert Bosch, Freescale Semiconductor, Kionix and VTI Technologies.

The newest inertial sensor to hit the market is the tri-axis accelerometer. In 2005, only a few companies manufactured them; but by early 2007, a dozen companies offered these sensors, and more companies will enter the market in the next year or two.

The ability to manufacture a sensor that can measure all three axes, for less than $1 in volume, is opening the door to some very creative applications. The most exciting is the Nintendo Wii™.

Currently, leading tri-axis accelerometer suppliers are Freescale Semiconductor, Hitachi and Kionix, but that will probably change fairly dramatically in the next couple of years.

Gyro Sensors

What makes a gyro sensor different from an accelerometer is that it measures rotational movement in the form of yaw (side to side rotation), pitch (up and down rotation) and roll. Think of the forward and backward, and side-to-side motion you experience on a roller coaster. If you've been on airplane when there's turbulence, you've also experienced yaw, pitch and roll.

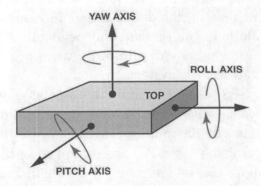

Rotational gyro movement. Copyright Analog Devices, Inc. All rights reserved.

The design of many gyros is just as complex as the accelerometer comb drives. But others are really, really simple. The gyro sold by Systron Donner Automotive is called a tuning fork gyro, because that's what it looks like—a tuning fork.

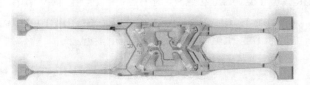

Photo courtesy of Systron Donner Automotive

Right now, the main application of gyros is in cars, as well as various military applications. But as the cost of these sensors decline, they're starting to find their way into consumer electronics, such as camcorders. In this case, they compensate for hand tremble, so you will never again take shaky, blurry videos!

Leading suppliers include BAE Systems, Robert Bosch, Honeywell and Systron Donner Automotive. However, there are a handful of firms who will challenge these companies and quite possibly take a leadership role in the next few years.

In some instances, companies combine an accelerometer (or two) with a gyro to create what's called an Inertial Measurement Unit (IMU). The purpose is to provide six-degrees-of-freedom sensing. In this respect, the device is able to monitor all types of linear *and* rotational movement, independently of each other: left/right, forward/backward, up/down, yaw, pitch and roll. This is the core of anti-rollover systems in cars.

If you add GPS (Global Positioning Systems) capability, then you have what's called an Inertial Navigation Unit, or INU, which is primarily in use by the military. If you've heard the term smart bomb, this is probably why. The integration of an INU makes the bomb much more accurate in terms of hitting its intended target; provided the coordinates entered into the system are correct.

Microfluidics

While most MEMS devices do indeed have moving parts, a meaningful segment does not: microfluidics. That is, MEMS devices that move fluid. Some of the microfluidics devices available include ink jet printer heads, pumps, valves and even needles. One category, Lab-on-a-chip, is a significant part of microfluidics, but I'm going to discuss that product in Chapter 4.

Ink Jet Printing

The concept of ink jet printing, as we know it today, is traceable to 1978, when Hewlett Packard (HP) began looking at the use of silicon micromachining to create disposable ink jet printing technology. The approach allowed for the creation of nozzles that were both extremely small and packed together—features required for high resolution and sharp contrast. Of course, it didn't happen overnight, as there was a lot of trial and error. However, in 1984, HP introduced the ThinkJet printer, the first to use (relatively) low-cost, batch-fabricated, disposable printheads.

Interestingly enough, Canon began developing ink jet technology at about the same that HP did, and the two apparently cross-licensed a lot of patents. In fact, HP is said to hold more than 9,000 patents relating to ink jet printing technologies.

This particular technology has certainly come a long way. HP's first ink jet cartridges had 12 nozzles that could print 1,000 drops in one second. Today's most advanced printheads have hundreds of nozzles and can print at rates of 18 million drops per second, with droplet sizes as small as one nanometer. But not all ink jet printing cartridges are MEMS.

There are two ink jet printing technologies: Continuous and Drop-on-Demand (DOD). DOD is by far the dominant approach, and consists of two types of cartridges: piezoelectric and MEMS.

The printhead of a piezoelectric (piezo) cartridge is permanent, not disposable, and uses tiny vibrating crystals to push droplets of ink out of the nozzles, which are typically stainless steel. The leading manufacturer of this type of printhead is Epson, and until recently, Spectra and Kodak.

Once sold to consumers, this approach is more typically used for commercial wide format printing; or at least it was. In mid 2006, Spectra (now renamed FUJIFILM Dimatix) switched to a hybrid piezo/MEMS printhead. HP followed suit with the same approach not too long after. The focus of these companies is industrial manufacturing, and printable electronics in particular. Here, nanomaterials of all kinds are playing an increasingly important role as the "ink."

The MEMS approach in DOD is called thermal bubble. Ink fills a cavity, which is then heated, creating bubbles (hence the name, thermal bubble). These bubbles of ink are then propelled out of the nozzle onto the paper. The empty cavity fills with ink and the process repeats itself thousands of times per *second*.

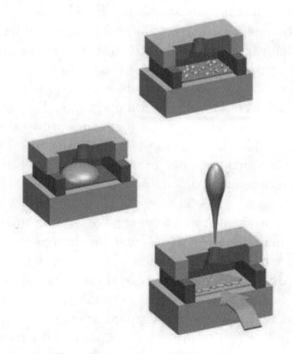

Illustrations courtesy of STMicroelectronics

Market leaders include Hewlett Packard, of course, as well as Canon, Lexmark and Dell, although Kodak introduced a MEMS printhead for consumer printers in early 2007.

Needles, Pumps, and Valves

Since needles, pumps and valves are important for moving fluid at the macro-scale, then why not at the micro-scale? Sure enough, microscopic needles, pumps and valves are indeed being manufactured for a variety of applications. Imagine this: MEMS needles so tiny that they're basically pain free; micromachined pumps small enough to be implanted under the skin to deliver insulin (see photo below); and silicon valves that efficiently move fluids throughout your car's various systems. These are all real.

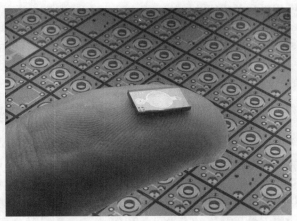

Array of MEMS pumps. Photo courtesy of Debiotech SA.

One of the most exciting microfluidic technologies I've come across is the capillary atomizer from Boehringer Ingelheim micro-Parts. Created for use in asthma inhalers, it's also being applied to consumer products. Called TruSpray®, the approach significantly reduces the need for propellants in aerosols.

It has a much finer diffusion than conventional spray products. The result is that a smaller can holds a more concentrated formulation. What makes this technology truly groundbreaking is that highly viscose products, like lotions, gels and waxes—which normally aren't sprayable—now are.

This innovation hasn't gone unnoticed in the packaging industry. In 2004, the TruSpray® package won the Red Dot Design Award. In 2005, it won the AEROBAL "Can of the Year" award and a silver Canmaker "Can of the Year" award, as well as the Worldstar award for Packaging Excellence.

Optical MEMS

The brief flash of sunlight off a reflective surface is something that you can't help but notice. It's become almost a cliché in movies, particularly during sword fighting scenes (where the glint of light on an exposed blade provides extra drama). But a signal mirror—a small, handheld mirror—is also an important piece of survival gear. Boy Scouts earn a merit badge learning how to use one, and they're part of many survival kits given to military personnel. Reflecting the sun to create a flash of light is far more efficient, and noticeable, than simply waving your arms for help.

This is the same basic concept used in next-generation televisions. Next time you go to the electronics store, take a look at the various options: liquid crystal and plasma probably come to mind first, but look a little closer for the DLP® logo. It's based on an optical MEMS device, which is essentially a tiny little mirror that reflects or moves light.

In the case of the Digital Light Processor (DLP), developed by Texas Instruments (TI), a chip less than one square inch in size contains up to 2.2 million individually moving mirrors to create the television image.

The DLP is, without a doubt, one of the most complex MEMS devices ever created. In late 2006, the company ran a series of television ads with the tagline "It's amazing, it's the mirrors," and amazing is certainly the right word.

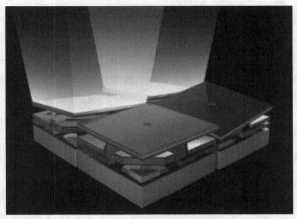

How MEMS mirrors move. Image courtesy Texas Instruments DLP Products®.

It took twenty years, but the effort certainly paid off. TI scientist Dr. Larry Hornbeck began work on the basic concept back in 1977. Ten years later, he built and tested the first DLP chip—at the time, it was generically referred to as a Digital Micromirror Device (DMD). In 1996, the first commercial product to rely on the chip to create images became available.

Texas Instruments initially focused their efforts on the emerging business projector market, recognizing that their technology could make this equipment lighter, and thus more portable. The impact was profound, to say the least. Today's smallest DLP projectors weigh about one pound (fitting comfortably in your hand), a far cry from the 50+ pound behemoths once called "portable" simply because you could lug them around school (or the office) on metal rolling carts.

In 2001, Texas Instruments shipped their one-millionth DLP sub-system. Just four years later, in 2006, the company reached a significant milestone by shipping its 10 millionth[5]. Having transformed the projector market, the company is finding great success in high-definition TVs and home theater systems.

At the complete opposite end of the spectrum, in terms of complexity, are single-mirror optical MEMS devices, like those from Microvision. These chips form the basis of wearable displays, and are also finding their way into cars and even barcode scanners. In fact, both Microvision and Intermec Technologies sell barcode scanners that use an optical MEMS device as the core technology. Somewhere in the middle are optical MEMS devices which are central to optical networking systems (to help switch light paths in optical fibers).

Another type of optical MEMS device is a deformable mirror, like those from Boston Micromachines. These compensate for variations in the optical effects that occur between an object and its image, such as those found in ophthalmology instruments and the telescopes used by astronomers.

Other MEMS Devices

The four categories above account for the vast majority of MEMS industry sales at this time, but there's so much more available, and in development. Products range from chemical/gas sensors, infrared and magnetic sensors, silicon microphones, a group of devices called RF MEMS, and all sorts of other things that are completely unique and defy categorization.

Chemical/Gas Sensors

While humans enjoy the scent of items such as cookies or wine, they've long sought ways to detect harmful substances, whether it's spoiled food or chemical weapons. The dog is known to have a highly evolved sense of smell and throughout history was helpful in tracking food. Today, they're used for search and rescue, as well as to identify drugs and other contraband, and even cancer[6]. But what about compounds that have no color, odor or taste?

The concept of "a canary in a coal mine" isn't folklore. Early on, miners used candles to detect the lack of oxygen (it would go out) or certain gases (the flame changed color). But this was hazardous, since the conditions of mines in and of themselves are potentially explosive. So, in some instances, canaries were put to use. This is because they react to harmful gases far more quickly than humans; if the bird stopped singing (because it either passed out or died), miners could take heed and get out—fast.

According to the British Broadcasting Corporation, birds were still in use in the United Kingdom as recently as the late 1980s[7].

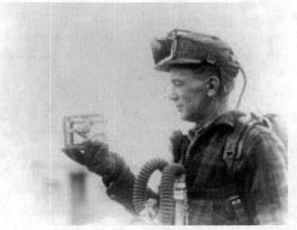

Coalminer with canary. Photo courtesy US Department of Labor, Mine Safety and Health Administration.

Today, a variety of electronic chemical and gas sensing technologies are available; but they aren't perfect. Considerable attention was paid to the development of such sensors after 9/11 for the detection of chemical and biological warfare agents. The "holy grail" is real-time detection of multiple compounds or chemical mixes, but the best systems today can generally only sense a single compound in a few minutes. In most situations, that's a few minutes too late.

Despite great strides in the research and development of such sensors, *Time Magazine* reported that U.S. troops apparently relied on chickens as their "canaries" during the early days of the Iraq war in 2003[8].

Still, the concept of an "electronic nose" is indeed a reality. However, despite the growing use of the term "nanosensor" in conjunction with such devices, many of these sensors today do not rely on either MEMS or nanotechnology—the few that do include lab-on-a-chip and cantilever sensors, as well as micro-spectrometers.

Micro-spectrometers are fairly new. Their larger counterpart, a spectrometer, is a bench-top system that measures the properties of light. Because of this, they can identify the unique fingerprint of chemicals, so they're incredibly accurate. This makes spectrometers especially useful in the detection of chemicals and gases; but they're very expensive and not at all portable.

The use of micromachined components (in this case, typically an optical MEMS device) means that such systems are now about the size of a lunch box. This is opening the door to applications that simply weren't possible before. The most talked about include those that are security-oriented, such as those used by military personnel, or at high-profile public events—even deployment in important infrastructure such as subway systems. But their usefulness in quantitative and purity analysis makes them ideal for material inspection and, thus, quality control. For example, the ability to differentiate between different polymers would make them useful in the production of nanocomposites.

Companies who currently manufacture and sell micro-spectrometers include AXSUN Technologies, Microsaic Systems, Owlstone Nanotech, Polychromix, Sionex and Thermo Electron.

Other firms are developing sensors to detect such compounds using approaches that rely on either a micromachined chip of some sort, nanomaterials, or both. However, only about half a dozen actually have products available today, a testament to the difficulty of developing this kind of sensor.

Microsens SA has an extensive product portfolio, with MEMS sensors able to measure oxygen (O_2), carbon monoxide (CO), carbon dioxide (CO_2), nitrogen oxide (NOx), methane (CH_4), butane (C_4H_{10}), ethyl alcohol (C_2H_5OH), and hydrogen (H_2).

Three other companies sell MEMS hydrogen sensors as well. Kebaili targets their sensor for use in conjunction with fuel cells. The sensor from Makel Engineering is qualified for use in space applications; and one from VIASPACE is also used in fuel cells.

MicroChemical Systems combines MEMS with nanoparticles for the detection of car emissions including ozone, carbon monoxide (CO), nitrogen oxide (NOx), nitrogen dioxide (NO_2), and hydrocarbons, as well as blood alcohol (ethanol). Another company with a gas sensor for detecting alcohol is Seju Engineering, who also uses their sensor to detect bad breath.

Infrared Sensors

When most people hear of infrared sensors, they probably think of night vision goggles—where people show up as a bright color against a black background. I, like many, incorrectly believed that this type of sensor measured heat. Instead, they're actually sensing wavelengths of radiation, which is an *effect* of heat. Technically, it's the movement of energy in the form of waves.

On a very hot day, have you ever noticed that the space just above a long stretch of highway looks wavy?

Early infrared sensors actually detected photons. In order to work, they needed to be cryogenically cooled (down to minus 200 hundred degrees Celsius), which limited their usefulness.

To get around this, Honeywell developed a new type of IR sensor, called a microbolometer, in the 1980s. The best part was that this technology didn't need to be cooled; which is why it's also referred to as an uncooled thermal (or IR) sensor. Honeywell licensed the technology to a number of companies and today, this type of sensor is sold by Electrophysics, FLIR Systems and others. They're actually used in airports to detect if arriving passengers have a fever, to prevent the possible spread of bird flu.

A second kind of MEMS-based infrared sensor is a thermopile, which is basically an array of thermocouples. A thermocouple converts thermal energy into electrical energy. This is different from a thermistor, which is an inexpensive temperature sensor. If you need to measure a high temperature, a wide temperature range, or need precise temperature measurements, then you use a thermopile. Companies who manufacture MEMS thermopiles include GE Sensing, Melexis, MEMSTech and Perkin Elmer.

More Cool Stuff

There's seemingly no end to the possibilities of creating three-dimensional structures in silicon (and other materials). Here are a few examples of other unique MEMS devices:

Fuel Cells

A handful of firms are creating tiny fuel cells (a unique new battery to power consumer electronics) leveraging MEMS fabrication techniques. The designs are fairly diverse, but micro fuel cells are essentially an array of tiny channels though which a flammable liquid, such as methanol, flows. The liquid reacts to a catalyst material that coats the channels, which results in a chemical reaction that generates power. Due to the small size of micro fuel cells, it's clear that nanoscale catalysts could further enhance these products. None are on the market just yet.

In the meantime, a number of MEMS sensors became commercially available in 2006, which are specifically for use in automotive fuel cells. These work the same way as micro fuel cells, but are much larger.

MEMS sensors for use in fuel cells include the Model FC6, a methanol density and chemical concentration sensor, from Integrated Sensing Systems; a flow sensor (for bubble detection and the measurement of flow rates) from Sensirion AG; and the HS-1000 from VIASENSOR, which monitors the level of humidity in hydrogen fuel cells.

Humidity Sensor

A humidity sensor from Hygrometrix measures relative humidity—ranging from 0 to 100 percent. What makes this sensor especially useful across a wide range of applications is that it works even after being frozen or totally immersed in water. There are a lot of products shipped under such conditions, such as food.

Magnetic Sensor

Honeywell, Yamaha and others sell a micromachined magnetic sensor. An interesting application is to combine it with a tri-axis accelerometer to create what's basically a magnetic compass. This is increasingly found in personal GPS systems.

Microphones

The future of microphones lies in silicon. Akustica, Infineon Technologies, Knowles Acoustics, MEMSTech and Sonion are at the forefront of this revolution. Millions of cell phones already use MEMS microphones.

RFID Tags

Alien Technology's radio frequency identification (RFID) tags are actually MEMS devices, despite being incorrectly identified as nanotechnology when they first hit the market. The confusion probably came about because the tags "self-assemble" after being manufactured, a quality often attributed to nanotechnology.

RF MEMS

This particular device category includes all sorts of components used to make electronics work more efficiently. End-uses include increasing the transmission efficiency of signals, such as the FBAR duplexers and filters from Avago Technologies; changing the flow of electrical currents, such as the switches from MEDER Electronics and Radant MEMS; converting current, such as the DC-DC converters from Enpirion; and creating electrical signals at a very precise frequency, such as the resonators/oscillators from Discera and SiTime. These companies, and their products, are just the beginning here—there's a lot more on the horizon.

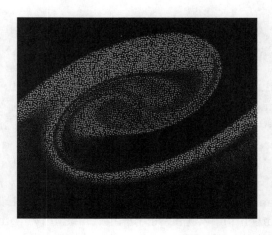

3 • NANOTECHNOLOGY

Now that tools are available so that we can see at the molecular level, scientists are finding all sorts of examples of nanotechnology throughout history (and nature): from Egyptian make-up and legendary steel, to stained glass windows and even rocks. The bottom line is that we're learning that nanotechnology is both a naturally occurring phenomena, and man-made.

Take rocks for example. Pink-colored nanofibers (100 nm to 500 nm) give rose quartz its unique color[9]. It's now known that opals consist of spheres ranging in size from 150 nm to 300 nm. The optical interference of these nanoparticles is what creates its iridescence—something the cosmetic industry is leveraging.

Another example of naturally-occurring nanotechnology is carbon black (known as lamp black for centuries). If you burn candles, or have an oil lamp, you're creating carbon black in your own home. It's technically produced by burning a hydrocarbon in a limited supply of air, and results in the fluffy, intensely black soot you see form around the rim of glass votives or oil lamps. Particles range in size from 8 to 300 nanometers. In ancient Egypt, China and India, they used it as an ink for writing and painting. Today, carbon black is not only found in the ink used to print newspapers, but it's also a major ingredient in tires.

Man-made examples of nanotechnology include the beautiful blue paint created by the Mayans, the brilliant red in Chinese porcelain and the deep, rich red found in medieval stained glass windows. But these were accidents, the result of varying materials and their chemical reactions; certainly the ancients had no knowledge of nanotechnology per se, or the capability to intentionally, or even knowingly, add nanoscale structures to their materials.

Metal nanoparticles are part of what made the Maya blue pigment so extraordinary[10]. In the case of the porcelain and stained glass, gold nanoparticles are the magic ingredient. At that size, they're not the yellow color we expect gold to be. Rather, when 30 nanometers in diameter, they absorb blue and yellow light, and reflect the color red instead.

One of the most exciting examples of nanotechnology in ancient times is the recent discovery of carbon nanotubes and nanowires in the highly-prized Damascus steel[11].

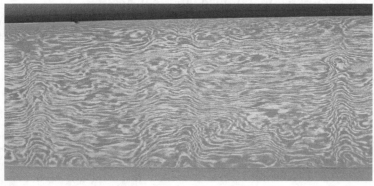

Close-up of Damascus steel. Photo courtesy Oriental-Arms Ltd, www.oriental-arms.il.

Legend has it that swords made of Damascus steel could cut through other swords (and even rock) without becoming dull, and could effortlessly slice a piece of silk in half as the material floated to the ground. The swords were also beautiful; a swirling moiré pattern, each one as unique as a fingerprint, made them instantly recognizable.

The production of swords and daggers made of this exceptional metal took place from roughly 1000 to 1700 AD; then the technique was inexplicably lost forever. It's hard to believe that the production process itself was forgotten. It's more reasonable to conclude that it was a lack of the specific materials used.

It's thought that the raw materials for the manufacture of these swords and daggers eventually ran out. If the replacement materials didn't duplicate the type and composition of the originals exactly, then the unique properties that came about as a result of combining them during the forging process wouldn't give subsequent swords the same qualities.

Today, of course, with the appropriate tools, we can maintain the consistency of raw materials at the nanoscale. This raises the exciting prospect that, perhaps now, we can indeed replicate this legendary steel once again.

The most important difference between naturally-occurring and man-made nanotechnology is our ability to design and produce nanoscale structures in whatever size desired, on a consistent, repeatable basis. In other words, it's all about quality control.

This is important, because particular sizes have specific physical properties, which can affect product performance. To that end, the most important part of man-made or "engineered" nanotechnology is the tools, the scanning tunneling microscopes and atomic force microscopy instruments, which allow for the ongoing discovery and production of nanoscale structures.

What makes nanotechnology tough to fully understand are the myriad of words used in conjunction with it. Common terms include nanomaterials, nanoparticles, nanostructures and a lot of nanoscale-something or another. They all basically describe the same thing, don't they?

For the most part, the terms nanomaterials and nanoparticles basically refer to any nanoscale material, which industry defines as having dimensions between one and 100 nanometers. However, as previously discussed, there are many examples of "nano-materials," "nanoparticles" and "nanoscale" referring to sub-micron materials as well (those ranging in size from 100 to 1,000 nanometers).

Add on top of that a dizzying array of product-specific categories: carbon nanotubes, dendrimers, fullerenes (aka buckyballs), nano-clays, nanocomposites, nanocrystals, nanofibers, nanopowders, nanostructures and quantum dots, and the world of nanotech-nology gets even more daunting. So, let's take a look at the various "nano" aspects of nanotechnology.

Carbon Nanotubes

Carbon nanotubes (CNT) are a cylindrical, tube-like arrange-ment of carbon atoms that are about 1 nanometer in diameter. If you unrolled one, you'd see a honeycomb-like structure. For those of you who like to build things, here's a hands-on way to under-stand their structure.

Next time you're at the hardware store, go to the fencing section and take a look at the chicken wire. It also has holes that are hexagonal in shape (like a honeycomb). If you cut a section and roll it into a tube, you have a structure that looks like a carbon nanotube—except a whole lot bigger, of course.

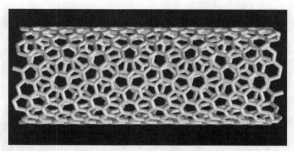

Image courtesy Jian-Min Zuo, University of Illinois Urbana-Champaign

What I just described is called a single walled carbon nanotube (SWNT). There are also multi walled carbon nanotubes (MWNT). In the case of the latter, as the name implies, rather than a single sheet rolled into a tube, you have multiple sheets rolled together; a little bit like the entire roll of chicken wire.

Carbon nanotubes are not manufactured individually; rather, they're "synthesized" via a number of techniques, including laser ablation (the process of removing material from a solid surface) and chemical vapor deposition (a way of creating thin films). As carbon nanotubes "grow," they naturally align themselves as a rope; a little bit like the individual strands of fiber that twist together to form yarn. In that respect, clusters of carbon nanotubes can end up looking a little bit like wall-to-wall carpeting.

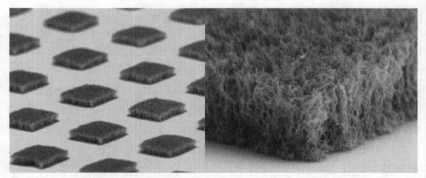

Credit is given to the University of California, Lawrence Livermore National Laboratory, and the Department of Energy, under whose auspices the work was performed.

47

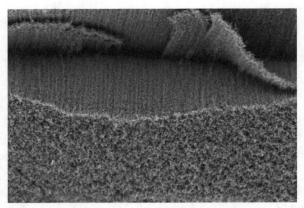

Thin-films of carbon nanotubes. Photo courtesy Pacific Northwest National Laboratory, William R. Wiley Environmental Molecular Sciences Laboratory.

Given the amount of press devoted to carbon nanotubes over the past several years, it's legitimate to ask: what's the big deal? And what makes them so special?

It turns out that carbon nanotubes are both incredibly strong—100 times stronger than steel—but much less dense, meaning they're a lot lighter. In fact, carbon nanotubes are 1/6th the weight of steel. They're also flexible, so they can bend fairly significantly without damage. Carbon nanotubes conduct electricity as well as copper; apply voltage and they can also emit light and/or heat.

If they sound like a virtual wonder material, well, they basically are; which is why researchers are so excited about the potential they offer (and have already demonstrated). For example, the company Nanocomp makes a yarn made entirely of carbon nanotubes for use as a conducting fiber or fabric.

Applications for which they're best suited right now are composite materials (basically polymers, or plastics, into which carbon nanotubes are added) and electronics (such as transistors). As you will see in Part 2 of this book, they're already found in products ranging from baseball bats to the fuel line of your car.

There are dozens of companies worldwide who produce carbon nanotubes, but only about 12 are major suppliers at this time; each of which have the capacity to produce *tons* of the material on an annual basis.

Leading Carbon Nanotube Suppliers			
Company	Location	Product	Brand
Arkema	France	MWNT	Graphistrength™
Bayer MaterialScience	Germany	MWNT	Baytubes™
Hyperion Catalysis	US	MWNT	FIBRIL™
ILJIN Nanotech	Korea	SWNT, MWNT	N/A
Mitsui & Co	Japan	SWNT, MWNT	AURUM™ CNT
Nanoamor	US	SWNT, MWNT	N/A
Nanocyl	Belgium	MWNT	N/A
Raymor	Canada	SWNT	N/A
Shenzhen Nano-Technologies Port	China	SWNT, MWNT	N/A
Showa Denko	Japan	N/A	N/A
Sun Nanotech	China	MWNT	Sunnano®
Unidym	US	SWNT, MWNT	Buckytubes

Source: Bourne Research LLC, 04/07

Mitsui is the market leader with an extensive background. In 2001, they founded Carbon Nanotech Research Institute (CNRI), which sells both SWNT and MWNT individually and in composites. In 2006, with Hodogaya Chemical, they formed a joint venture focused on MWNT called Nano Carbon Technologies. Mitsui Chemicals also recently launched a new grade of nano-composite called AURUM™ CNT in cooperation with Hyperion Catalysis, who's actually a competitor.

Following is an example of the distribution chain that can be involved: Arkema supplies their carbon nanotubes to both Nanoledge and Zyvex. Zyvex, in turn, adds them to a polymer, then supplies this nanocomposite to Easton Sports, who manufactures bike components with it; both for themselves and for other bike manufacturers.

Dendrimers

A dendrimer is a synthetic, three-dimensional, star-shaped molecule that can be as small as three or four nanometers in diameter. In some respects, it looks a bit like a snowflake.

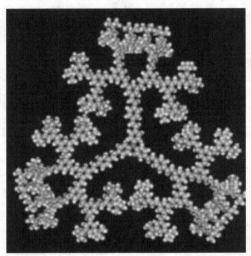

Close-up of a dendrimer. Photo courtesy of Cambridge DisplayTechnologies.

Some of the unique properties of dendrimers include:

- Low viscosity—Dendrimers are less resistant to flow, like milk, as opposed to mashed potatoes, which are highly viscose in comparison.
- High solubility—Dendrimers can easily dissolve in water.
- High reactivity—This is the ability to change when combined with another substance; highly reactive substances may explode.
- Low compressibility—The volume of dendrimers won't decrease much under increased pressure.

Because of these properties, dendrimers can make materials more water resistant and adhere better to surfaces like glass, plastic and metal, as well as speed up curing (ie. drying). In this respect, it makes sense that the Priostar™ dendrimers from Dendritic Nanotechnologies and the PAMAM dendrimers from Dendritech are being targeted for use in ink jet inks and toners.

Their reactivity is useful to Cambridge Display Technology, who is using dendrimers to create next-generation displays comprised of polymer-based light emitting diodes (PLED). Dendrimers are also finding use in medicine to improve the delivery of drugs into the body.

Fullerenes (aka Buckyballs)

Fullerenes (formally called buckminsterfullerenes and often referred to as buckyballs) are molecular clusters of pure carbon which look a lot like soccer balls. In terms of structure, they're very similar to carbon nanotubes, except that they are round, rather than tube-shaped.

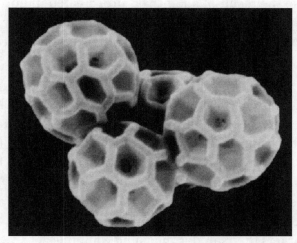

DNA buckyballs. Photo courtesy of Dan Luo, Cornell University.

Fullerenes are extremely hard, can withstand high temperature and pressure (they spring back to shape when compressed), and also bounce. As a result, some of their earliest applications were as a composite material for use in things like sporting goods. Coatings and films are also strong application areas.

The fact that fullerenes are hollow is one of their most unique properties. Because of this, researchers are very interested in their potential use in all sorts of medical applications, ranging from MRI (magnetic resonance imaging) agents, to drug delivery vehicles—all by "filling" them with various materials.

Several dozen companies produce fullerenes, many of whom also produce carbon nanotubes. However, two companies really stand out in terms of production capacity: Frontier Carbon and Fullerene International.

Frontier Carbon is the result of a joint venture created in 2001 between Mitsubishi Corporation and Mitsubishi Chemical. The company claims it can make 40 tons of fullerenes a year and plans to expand that capacity to 1,500 tons per year. Fullerene International is also the result of a joint venture, created in 2001 between three companies: Mitsubishi, Materials and Electrochemical Research (MER), and Research Corporation Technologies.

Nanoclays

Nanoclays are basically what the name implies: clay at the nanoscale. Three companies produce montmorrillonite; part of the smectite group of clays, which also includes talc (the main ingredient in baby powder). This particular clay has found use throughout the ages in cosmetics and for medicinal purposes. Nanocor sells their nanoclay via the brand name Nanomer®; Southern Clay Products calls their product Cloisite®; and Süd-Chemie markets theirs under the name Nanofil®.

Halloysite, which is part of the kaolite group of clays, is produced by a company called NanoClay and Technologies. This type of clay is generally used in porcelain, bone and fine china. But their clay differs from other halloysite clays in that it has a naturally occurring nanotube-like structure.

Nanoclays aren't generally sold as a stand-alone product; rather, they are incorporated into a polymer to create a plastic composite instead. The resulting material is lighter, stiffer, less porous and more scratch-resistant and paintable than current plastic compositess.

Other properties include better flame retardance, better electrical conductance, maintaining shape during temperature fluctuations and being less brittle in cold weather. All of these are especially important to the automotive industry. Take a look at your car, sport utility vehicle or truck and all of the plastic parts on the exterior, such as side-view mirror casings or step assists. For the food industry, the use of such a material results in improved shelf-life, shipping and product stability. Just think of the clear plastic films that cover nearly all of the food sold.

Nanoclay-based Composites

A composite is made up of two components: a matrix, which is basically the base material, and the filler, which is mixed into the matrix to make it stronger. Think of it a little bit like water and instant potato flakes. The dried flakes, when added to the water, make a material (mashed potatoes), which is a lot denser than just water alone. Changing the ratio of matrix and filler can change the consistency, and properties, of the end product.

So, with current plastics, the matrix is typically resin or nylon, and the filler is generally talc or glass. Unfortunately, those fillers result in cloudy, brittle plastic. We already know that particles can become transparent at the nanoscale, so using nanoclay doesn't make plastic cloudy. In addition, because of the greater surface area, less filler is needed, so the plastic remains flexible, in addition to the other qualities discussed above. The plastic's properties can be adjusted simply by changing the size and amount of particles used.

Clay-based nanocomposites are perhaps one of the most widely used nanomaterial today, with dozens of companies offering and/or developing such products. They can be found in all sorts of plastic parts in cars, lawn and garden equipment, the plastic films and bottles used to package food, and construction items such as siding, fencing and doors, as well as things like stadium seats and big plastic containers—virtually any item made of plastic today.

Here are some of the leading firms and a hint of where we can find each of their products.

- Basell Polyolefins' thermoplastic nanocomposite were part of the step-assists on the 2001 GM minivans. They used nanoclays from Southern Clay.

- BASF offers two products: Ultradur® High Speed, whose nanoparticles range in size from 50 nm to 300 nm, and COL.9®, for use in exterior paint and coatings.

- Bayer is incorporating nanoclays from Nanocor to create see-through films (think plastic wrap on food). They also produce a flame-retardant nanocomposite, and through its GE Bayer Silicones joint venture, have a scratch-proof and soil-repellent coating using a clay-based nanocomposite.

- ColorMatrix offers Imperm® for use in multilayer bottles (for a wide range of carbonated beverages), food films and containers, as well as coated paper cartons.

- Du Pont is currently developing a line of thermoplastic nanocomposites called DNM—it is expected to become commercially available in mid 2007.

- Honeywell offers Aegis™ NC, for film and paper coatings, and Aegis™ OX, for plastic beer bottles. Yes, *plastic* beer bottles. They use nanoclays from Nanocor.

- NaturalNano is developing the nanocomposite Pleximer™, which uses nanoclays from NanoClay and Technologies. It is expected to become commercially available sometime in late 2007.

- Noble Polymers offers three clay-based nanocomposites: Forte™ (for use by the automotive industry), Ecobarrier™ (for use as a sound barrier in low heat environments), and Regis™ (for high-strength automotive applications).

- Nycoa has two nanocomposites: nanoTuff™ (for use where cold weather is a factor) and nanoSEAL™ (for automotive fuel systems).

- PolyOne's Nanoblend™ is used in automotive, packaging, construction, and many other applications. They use nanoclays from Nanocor.

- SolVin is a joint venture between Solvay and BASF. Their product, NanoVin®, is used in auto body panels and artificial leather.

Nanofibers

Nanofibers are basically what the name implies: fibers at the nanoscale. They are created by a process called electrospinning, which is basically this: a needle is filled with a liquid polymer, electricity is applied to pull out the material in a continuous stream and then it's whipped around really fast so that the stream of material can be stretched into nanometer dimensions. The end result is a web of tiny fibers. It's a little like creating cotton candy, but at the nanoscale. So, next time you're at a fair, go take a closer look at the cotton candy machine.

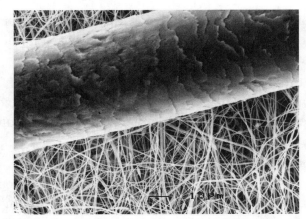

Nanofibers and a human hair. Photo courtesy of eSpin Technologies.

Nanofibers are spun for use as both textiles and membranes—that is, woven and non-woven materials. Most products on the market today are membranes for the filtration of air and liquid. Japan Vilene's nanofiber is used as a separator in batteries. Koch offers nanofibers for the filtration of liquids in industrial applications, such as food and textile processing.

Donaldson offers two products for industrial air filtration and pollution control: Ultra-Web® is for dust collection and Spider-Web® is for air filtration in gas turbines. Their Endurance™ air filters are for use in heavy-duty engines.

Two companies are well-known for their development of nanofibers for woven textiles, and both are Japanese. Toray Industries has been working for years on the development of both nanofibers and nano-based fiber coatings.

One of the most intriguing fibers is from Teijin Fiber Corporation. MORPHOTEX® is a very unique fiber that produces an iridescent effect. It is comprised of 61 layers of polyester and nylon fibers, each of which are just a few nanometers thick, and each with a different refractive index. This basically means that, depending on its thickness, each layer is some variation of red, blue, green or yellow. Viewing angle and light intensity also play a role in what color you see. Even better, since it doesn't rely on any dyes or pigments, its colors won't fade.

The company is targeting textiles, paint and cosmetics as key applications. Fibers in cosmetics? It's not as far-fetched as you might think. Fibers are already used in mascara to help thicken and lengthen lashes; they can also help to strengthen nails via nail polish. The iridescent quality of this fiber would certainly be a sought-after effect in such cosmetics. As for paint—think automobiles. The use of such a fiber could certainly create unique paints for cars and trucks.

Nanoparticles

Nanoparticles are available commercially in the form of dry powders, coatings, films and liquid dispersions. The latter is obtained by combining nanoparticles with a liquid to form a suspension or paste.

As indicated at the beginning of this chapter, "engineered" nanoparticles are created with specific properties—generally size— to meet the specific need of a particular application. The most common nanoparticles are simple metal oxides:

- Aluminum oxide (Al_2O_3)—Also known as alumina, aluminum oxide is a great insulator, so it is often used in electronic and magnetic coatings, and as a component in ceramics. Its primary use is in chemical-mechanical planarization (CMP) slurries, which are used in the production of semiconductors.

- Cerium oxide (CeO_2)—Also known as ceria, cerium oxide is used in ceramics and to polish glass, and is finding application in fuel cells.

- Iron oxide (Fe_3O_4 and Fe_2O_3)—There are 16 different iron oxides. Uses include ceramic glazes (where exposure to high temperatures produces the colors you see on pottery) and cosmetics.

- Silicon dioxide (SiO_2)—Also known as silica, silicon dioxide is the primary ingredient in the production of glass, cement, ceramics (like pottery) and optical fibers. It's also a food additive, and is used to improve the flow of powdered food and to absorb water.

- Titanium dioxide (TiO_2)—Also known as titania, it is primarily used as a white pigment in paints, coatings, plastics, papers, ink, food and toothpaste. Its UV resistant properties are especially useful in plastics.

- Zinc oxide (ZnO)—Not quite as opaque as titanium dioxide, zinc oxide is used as a white pigment in paint and coatings for paper. It is the primary ingredient (in combination with iron oxide) in calamine lotion. Because zinc oxide reflects both UVA and UVB rays, it is widely used as a sunscreen.

- Zirconium dioxide (ZrO_2)—Also known as zirconia, zirconium dioxide is used in ceramics to improve their toughness, as well as resistance to fracture and chipping.

Nanoparticles are becoming increasingly important for use as catalysts of all kinds, scratch-resistance coatings and color pigments. In the case of the latter, the sky is virtually the limit.

Nanoparticle-based pigments (generally iron oxides) are currently used to give color to things like rubber latex, non-woven fabrics, paper coatings, lumber marking, artists' colors and architectural paints. They are already found on kettle grills, stoves, and washers and dryers, as well as asphalt roofing shingles and even glazing products used to decorate floor tiles and dinnerware. And, of course, cosmetics and personal care products are a key end-use.

There are countless companies manufacturing nanoparticles of all sorts. Some focus on just a few, while others can manufacture nearly every known compound at the nanoscale. Following are some of the leading companies in nanoparticle commercialization.

- American Elements offers a line called Nanometal™ (which includes about 100 different elements) and Z-Mite™, a zinc oxide available in diameters ranging from 10 to 200 nm.

- BASF offers Z-COTE® MAX, which they describe as a microfine zinc oxide ultraviolet (UV) light absorber. The nanoparticles are supplied to them by Nanophase.

- Bayer offers Dispercoll® S, a silica gel dispersion for use in water-based adhesives like those used to bond foam, laminate wood and even hold together the pieces of shoes.

- Degussa offers several different lines of nanoparticles: AdNano® Zinc Oxide (for food packaging, coatings and personal care), AdNano® Ceria (for CMP, catalysts, fuels cells and more), AdNano® Indium Tin Oxide ITO (to prevent static on plastic and painted surfaces) and AdNano® MagSilica (for things like adhesives).

- Engelhard, now part of BASF, offers the most comprehensive family of nanoparticles today. They sell catalysts for cars and petroleum refining (HiQ®, HiTemp™, Flex-Tec™, and NaphthaMax®), and an extensive range of color effect-pigments for automotive exteriors, cosmetics, plastics, coatings and inks. Specific applications range from coatings on seeds, appliances and leather, to toys, sporting goods and textiles.

- Nanophase offers NanoArc® (bismuth oxide, copper oxide and iron oxide), NanoDur® (Aluminum oxide), NanoGard® (zinc oxide), NanoShield® (zinc oxide), and NanoTek® (aluminum oxide, antimony tin oxide, indium tin oxide, tin oxide and zinc oxide).

- QinetiQ currently offers Tesimox™ oxides (alumina, zirconia, yttria, zinc oxide, cerium oxide and titanium oxide), Tesimet™ metals (aluminum, copper, nickel, tungsten, and silver) and Tesmide™ metal carbides and nitrides.

Nanosilver

One of the most talked about nanomaterials is silver nanoparticles. Silver suddenly seems to be everywhere, from clothes to washing machines and pretty much anything in between. You might also recognize the term nanosilver, which refers to any use of silver at the nanoscale. So, what's the big deal?

The antibacterial properties of silver are well known. Some bacteria, of course, can make you sick; silver can kill such germs very quickly. And since bacteria are what create smell, the use of silver eliminates odor. The Greeks and Romans added silver coins to vessels holding water (and even used silver containers). It's said that during the plague, wealthy families ate with silverware to protect themselves—that puts a whole new spin on "born with a silver spoon in one's mouth" doesn't it? And pioneers in the U.S. apparently placed silver coins in milk jugs and wooden water casks to keep those liquids fresher longer.

The concept isn't new; just the form. Today, silver is being used in various ways, including nanoparticles, which began generating a lot of controversy in early 2006. So much so that in October

2006, the US Environmental Protection Agency announced that consumer products which promote the use of silver "for the purpose of killing microbial pests" will be regulated as a pesticide and are thus subject to registration requirements under the Federal Insecticide, Fungicide & Rodenticide Act.

It appears that at least some of the impetus behind this was the SilverCare washing machine from Samsung, which releases silver ions into clothes during the rinse cycle. A number of organizations raised concerns about the impact of silver nanoparticles subsequently released into the environment. But this brings up a really important question: are ions nanoparticles?

Let's start with the basic building blocks of life: atoms. Atoms are about one-third of a nanometer in diameter. Two or more atoms are what make up a molecule, which range in size from a few angstrom to several dozen angstrom. One angstrom is one-tenth of a nanometer. An ion is a charged atom or molecule.

Since some describe nanotechnology as the manipulation of atoms and molecules, does this mean that something *smaller* than 1 nanometer is a nanoparticle? This goes back to the difference between a form of measurement and the precise manufacturing of something. Like red blood cells and bacteria, ions already exist. They might be nanoscale, but they are not man-made.

This is important, since the leading supplier of silver in an ever growing list of products—Agion Technologies—uses ions packed within zeolites.

Zeolites look a little bit like a sugar cube, have a honeycomb-like structure, and are typically about one micron in size. That alone is far too big to be considered a nanoparticle. But the voids, or pores, of the zeolite, are just a few angstroms in diameter, or about half a nanometer; and those contain silver ions.

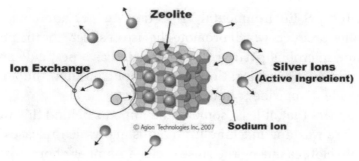

How a zeolite works. Image courtesy of Agion Technologies.

How do they work? Ambient air contains sodium (or salt) ions, and they basically switch places with the silver ions. So the zeolite slowly releases silver ions into the environment to kill whatever bacteria are present.

Agion Technologies' product clearly doesn't fit within the scope of nanoparticles. The delivery vehicle is microscale; if it were sub-micron, than that might be another story. The use of ions excludes them as well.

Even more important, it's registered with the EPA for use in a wide variety of applications ranging from food and water contact, to HVAC and building products, appliances, textiles, cosmetics and personal products. In addition, it's also approved by the US Food and Drug Administration (FDA) for some applications.

There is a second product on the market that's also frequently referred to as nanosilver, but isn't. Noble Fiber Technologies manufactures X-STATIC, a fiber which is coated with silver. This has actually been in the market for quite some time, and the coating method is decades old. If the coating were nano-scale, then the case could be made to call it nanotechnology, but at this point, it isn't. X-STATIC is also EPA-registered.

It's important to describe the above technologies in some detail, since these two approaches make up the bulk of silver-embedded products on the market today. The bottom line is, just because you see something with silver in it (to kill bacteria or control odor), that doesn't necessarily mean that nanoparticles are being used.

To a certain extent, Samsung's use of the word "Nano Technology" in conjunction with silver ions blurred the distinction between what is, and isn't, nanotechnology. And it illustrates how some manufacturers simply used the terminology for marketing.

As for those who are indeed using a true nanoparticle approach, there are about a dozen companies who do sell silver nanoparticles (some of which are noted earlier), but for most of them, their primary application is semiconductor manufacturing. A few are focused exclusively on the medical market, in which case, their products must receive approval from the U.S. Food and Drug Administration; some already have.

At this time, I know of three companies selling silver nanoparticles for use in consumer products: NanoHorizons (whose focus is textiles), Ciba Specialty Chemicals (who actually gets their silver nanoparticles from a company called Bio-Gate) and CMI Enterprises (whose focus is vinyl fabrics). Some of the applications in which their products can be found will be discussed in subsequent chapters.

Other Nanostructures

There are two other interesting nanoscale products that I would like to briefly touch on: aerogels and quantum dots.

Aerogels

One of the lightest materials in the world, aerogels are three times lighter than air, and 4,000 times stronger than their own weight. Sometimes called frozen smoke, because that's sort of what it looks like, aerogels were first developed in the early 1930s. They can be made of a number of different materials, but silica is by far the most common.

What makes aerogels unique is the fact that they are comprised of about 95 percent air; this is what gives them their translucent "frozen smoke" appearance. The key here is the fact that the "pores" of air are nanoscale. Structurally, aerogels are similar to sponges, and feel like Styrofoam. The best description I know of is that they are very similar to the green foam used by florists. You can find that foam in craft stores, take a look.

Why are aerogels special? As the photo illustrates so well, they have remarkable insulating properties—under any other circumstances, those crayons would be a melted mess. Aerogels basically block all three types of heat transfer: convection (despite being mostly air, air can't circulate through it), conduction (it doesn't conduct heat well), and radiation (it absorbs infrared heat).

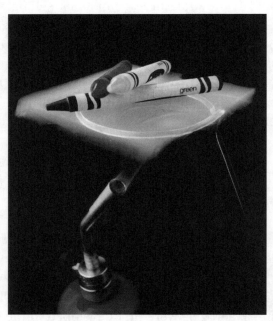

Aerogel protecting crayons. Photo courtesy of NASA Jet Propulsion Laboratory.

Because of these insulating qualities, they are already playing a role in windows, home appliances and even footwear. Companies who produce this unique material for these kinds of applications include Aspen Aerogels and Cabot Corporation.

Interestingly, Dow Corning now sells two aerogel-based ingredients for use in cosmetics. The products are microscale beads of aerogel material; so the microbeads themselves are made up of nanoscale pores of air. Properties that make them useful in this kind of application are their ability to absorb oil and the fact that aerogels are a good thickening agent. In addition, they also provide what is called a "soft focus effect" so that fine lines and wrinkles aren't so noticeable. I'm all for that!

Quantum Dots

Also called a nanocrystal, quantum dots are a unique semi-conductor-like material; they're basically a 1 nanometer piece of a silicon wafer. They have unique optical and electronic properties, and glow, or fluoresce, when shining blue or ultraviolet light on them. When that happens, they can emit bright light in an extensive range of colors.

Despite this property, electronics are not the primary focus. Rather, the two companies who produce quantum dots, Evident Technologies (with their EviDots™) and Invitrogen (via their QDOts), are generally targeting biomedical applications. Why? The unique light-emitting property of quantum dots means that life science researchers can conduct experiments and studies for longer periods of time than they can with other materials.

It's kind of fun to do the impossible.

—*Walt Disney*

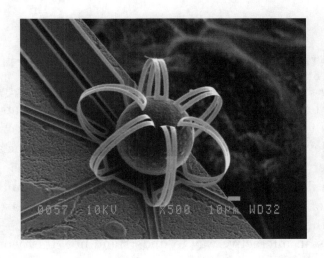

4 • NEMS
(NANOELECTROMECHANICAL SYSTEMS)

NanoElectroMechanical Systems are the ultimate convergence of nanotechnology and MEMS. That is, both approaches are required. Generally, a MEMS device forms the basic underlying technological platform, with some sort of nanomaterial or nano-structure coming into play as a key component.

An imaginative example of a NEMS device is the nanoguitar built by researchers at Cornell University in 1998. A replica of the Fender Stratocaster, the guitar is 10 microns long, but the strings are just 50 nanometers wide. Fabricated using MEMS micro-machining techniques, it illustrates how both MEMS and nanoscale structures are essential to the overall device. You can see a photo of the guitar at the beginning of Chapter 10.

The best known NEMS devices are cantilevers (the basis for one of the most important tools in the research and development of nanotechnology), as well as semiconductor testing, and a really unique product called lab-on-a-chip.

67

Atomic Force Microscopes (AFM)

The best example of NEMS at work is the Atomic Force Microscope (AFM). This is an instrument that uses tiny tips attached to the end of a micromachined cantilever to create images of the hills and valleys of any conducting or non-conducting surface. The cantilever itself looks (and acts) very much like a diving board. The cantilever and tip combined remind me of a microscopic version of the arm and needle of a record player (please tell me I'm not the only one who actually remembers those).

Here's an interactive way to understand how they work. Place the flat part of a tack on the end of your index finger, so that it covers the padded area where your fingerprint is. This will look a lot like the basic AFM structure. Now, lightly drag or tap the pointed tip across your kitchen counter—if you were connected to AFM imaging software, it would re-create a smooth, flat surface. If you lightly dragged your finger across something with texture, such as a basketball, then the image created would be a round shape with lots of tiny, regularly spaced indentations. Just like the surface of a basketball.

AFM is ideal for characterizing nanoparticles and nanoscale structures, and provides both qualitative and quantitative information on size, as well as surface area and texture—from individual particles to groups of particles.

Because the tip itself ranges in size from just a few nanometers to a few microns wide, it is able to image anything from 1 nanometer to several microns. Even better, an AFM can image things immersed in liquid. All of this takes place in just a few minutes.

Atomic force microscopes play a very important role in the inspection of semiconductor wafers, but it wouldn't be a stretch to say that this tool revolutionized nanotechnology, and is vital for its research, development and commercialization. The ability to image, measure and manipulate nanoscale materials is critical, and AFM does just that. This is the core of nanoscience—or the study of things at the nanoscale. Creation of 3D imagery takes place via the use of a laser.

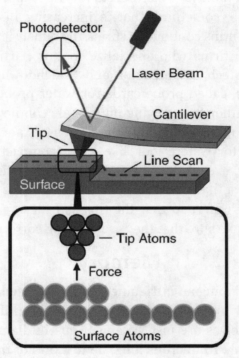

How an AFM works. Diagram courtesy of Agilent Technologies, Inc.

The best-known supplier of AFM tools is Agilent Technologies, who solidified their position in 2006 with the acquisition of Molecular Imaging. Other leading companies include Asylum Research, Nanosurf, Novascan Technologies, Pacific Nanotechnology and Veeco Instruments.

Not all of these companies manufacture their own cantilevers/tips, and there is quite an array to choose from, depending on the need. They range from super sharp to tipless, and even have diamond or magnetic coatings. Top suppliers of these elements include BudgetSensors, NanoSensors and Olympus.

I mentioned the use of cantilevers for the inspection and test of semiconductors, something that is increasing in importance as semiconductor firms continue to shrink the dimensions of integrated circuits. Three firms who specialize in this particular area are Cascade Microtech, FormFactor and Touchdown Technologies. Their products, called probe cards (or wafer probes), differ from AFM in that rather than relying on a single cantilever and tip, the cards contain an array of many—thousands in some cases.

Semiconductor wafers look like a big compact disc. A probe card is similar, except that it has a lot of tiny structures sticking out of it—almost like a microcopic cheese grater. It's placed over a semiconductor wafer, so that the tips can then touch the ICs on the wafer to make sure that they are working correctly.

Memory

IBM is developing an intriguing memory technology—called the Millipede—which also relies on an array of cantilevers. Because the tips themselves are just 40 angstroms in diameter, and each cantilever is only 10 microns long, up to 1,000 of these tips can fit into an area just three millimeters square.

What makes this memory technology even more unique is that it uses a 50 nanometer layer of polymer, rather than silicon, as the substrate. The tips write data by heating up and then creating an indentation in the polymer. They read data by measuring temperature; the tip is cooler when it is in the indentation versus when it's not. The entire concept is fascinating.

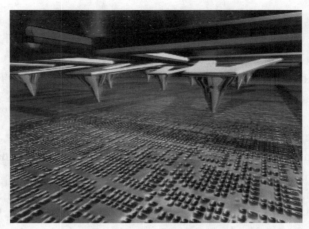

Reprint courtesy of International Business Machines Corporation
Copyright 2007 © International Business Machines Corporation

As they read and write data, this array of a thousand tips look a little bit like someone playing piano, or typing on a keyboard. Of course, this is still very much in development, but it's certainly closer to commercialization than it was a decade ago. Whether it will ever actually make it to market is a big question. But IBM isn't alone. A start-up by the name of Nanochip is also working on a memory chip based on a similar approach.

Sensors

Some biological and chemical sensors now fall under the NEMS umbrella due to their use of an array of cantilevers. In this case, they look a little bit like a comb. Because of the way they work, they remind me of a row of diving boards, each with a nanoscale coating of various materials. The principle is fairly basic and results in a highly sensitive biological or chemical sensor.

The material used to coat each cantilever recognizes and binds to whatever it is you want to detect. As a result, there is an infinitesimal change to its mass, or weight, so the cantilever bends

71

(hence its resemblance to a diving board). An array of lasers illuminates the cantilevers, and so when they bend, the system notes the change in the light pattern.

Oak Ridge National Laboratory created one of the first such sensors back in the 1990s, and subsequently licensed it to a number of companies, including Sense Holdings, who intends to use it for the detection of explosives.

What about nanosensors? The cantilever-based sensors just discussed are frequently called nanosensors. And there are a few firms (which I mentioned in Chapter 2) who are combining MEMS chips with nanomaterials. I have also noticed that some lab-on-a-chip devices, particularly those for industrial sensing, are more frequently being referred to as nanosensors as well.

Lab-on-a-Chip

If you're a Star Trek fan (the original television series in particular), then you're familiar with a medical tool called the "Tri-Corder," which could diagnose a patient's condition in seconds. One simply waved a small, hand-held device about the size of a thumb drive over the patient (as it flashed lights and made very scientific-sounding noises while collecting the necessary data). It was then placed into a device about the size of a small notebook so the doctor could read the results.

The basic concept is already in use in hospitals today, via the use of a device called lab-on-a-chip. Although, rather than waving the device over the patient, a few drops of blood are needed.

Lab-on-a-chip is part of a broader product category called bio-chips. Biochips are also a generic umbrella term for all of the chips now used in drug discovery and point-of-care diagnostics. But biochips (also called microarrays) are distinctly different from lab-on-a-chip, even though lab-on-a-chip is now considered a type of biochip. I know this is confusing, but stay with me here.

Biochips/microarrays are basically produced by ink jet printing (or screen printing) biological material onto glass. Lab-on-a-chip requires etching or embossing channels within a substrate of some sort. So, the difference is something that uses MEMS fabrication (lab-on-a-chip), versus a product that doesn't (biochips). Interestingly enough, in many cases, MEMS ink jet printheads are now used to create today's biochips.

Why is the distinction important? The capabilities of lab-on-a-chip are much broader than biochips.

With a biochip, DNA is simply attached to glass slides. This makes them useful in gene-based research (generally called gene expression). Researchers utilize them to study how genes react under certain conditions or to detect the mutations that cause certain genetic diseases.

Lab-on-a-chip prepares and processes liquid samples so you can test for specific things, like whether you are having a heart attack or if a dangerous chemical is present in water. But lab-on-a-chip is also used for gene expression too.

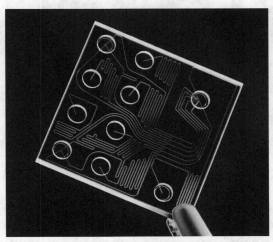

A simple lab-on-a-chip. © *Agilent Technologies, Inc. 2007. Reproduced with Permission, Courtesy of Agilent Technologies, Inc.*

The core of lab-on-a-chip is microfluidics—the ability to move, mix and control extremely small amounts of fluid. Some of these chips are very simple, consisting of just a few channels. Others are incredibly complex, with arrays of channels, pumps and valves etched or embossed into plastic, glass or silicon.

Where does the nanotechnology angle come in? The fact that the samples used are generally measured in nanoliters, has led some to equate lab-on-a-chip with nanotechnology. However, a few of the chips themselves do use materials in their construction, such as gold, that are just nanometers thick.

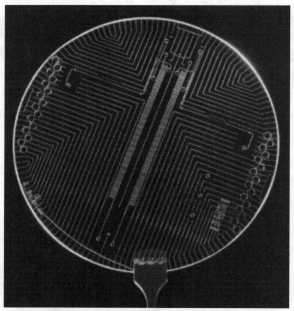

Copyright 2007 © National Academy of Sciences, U.S.A.[12]

One of the biggest challenges with these devices is the fact that liquid has completely different properties at the micro scale. Water in a drinking glass moves freely and can be splashed about.

In a lab-on-a-chip device, however, it has long been known that water takes on a property called "laminar flow." That is, it moves really slowly and smoothly, like lava oozing out from a volcano, or pouring molasses from a jar. Plus, when you're dealing with biological material, such as blood, then there is the issue of getting cells to move through the channels, rather than clogging them up.

The development of lab-on-a-chip came about as a result of the need for life science researchers to reduce the amount of materials used for tests, increase throughput (the number of tests conducted at any given time), integrate multiple steps into a single step, reduce cross-contamination and lower overall research costs. In addition, laboratory analysis is time consuming.

Lab-on-a-chip not only offers much faster assay times (the amount of time it takes for a test to run through completion), but they use much smaller samples and reagent materials (the chemicals used to create reactions). They have also reduced the number of steps required during the assay process. Since they are disposable, cross-contamination is greatly lessened, as is cost.

Due to these properties, most of the companies focused their development of lab-on-a-chip for use by researchers involved in genomics (research about the human gene) and the discovery and development of new drugs. These chips, which work with DNA, cost hundreds of dollars, but they have proven themselves very useful in genomics research. This is because they can conduct polymerase chain reaction (PCR), a key to gene expression, far faster than previous technologies. In this respect, lab-on-a-chip is driving the development of personalized medicine—drugs that are created for specific types of cancer, for example, rather than cancer as a whole.

Despite the focus on life science research, early on a couple of companies looked elsewhere: point-of-care (POC) diagnostics. POC diagnostics allows doctors in emergency rooms to obtain test results for important blood parameters (such as blood gases, electrolytes, chemistries, coagulation and hematology)—in many cases, in less than a minute or two.

Beyond basic blood profiling, some really interesting specialized tests have emerged in the past few years. Some, such as those from Biosite Diagnostics, detect what are called cardiac markers; proteins in the blood that indicate whether you are having a heart attack. Rather than drawing blood and waiting several hours for the results, the results come back in minutes, so treatment can begin much sooner. Even better, they are inserted into and read by portable, hand-held units about the same size as a cordless phone handset or a really large TV remote.

A few years ago a third segment began to emerge, something I refer to as clinical diagnostics. Here, the DNA capabilities of life science research chips are combined with the rapid detection capabilities of POC diagnostics to create chips that can conduct unique DNA-based tests. Targeted areas include things like breast cancer, bird flu and E coli. The common thread is that with these kinds of tests, results are needed in minutes, but trimming the time it takes to get results from weeks to days can make a real difference in diagnosis and treatment.

Lab-on-a-chip is also beginning to move beyond medicine. Actually, a lot of really interesting applications have popped up over the years, such as identifying genetically modified crops, examining forensics/crime scene evidence, detection of biological and chemical warfare agents, and even food analysis.

Sensicore uses lab-on-a-chip technology to monitor water quality in municipal water treatment plants. Their WaterPOINT system can provide more than a dozen chemical measurements, with a single, handheld unit, in just a few minutes. Previously, the wait time was anywhere from an hour to several days for results. With increased concern about the safety of water supplies, this type of product is very timely. As with POC, the reader unit is a small, portable, handheld device.

About six companies got the whole lab-on-a-chip segment started in the early 1990s, nearly all of whom subsequently went public just a few years later. Since then, dozens of companies have joined them in their quest, ranging from small start-ups to large multinationals.

But, the basic hurdles remain; and so at this time, only about ten companies actually have products on the market today.

Leading Lab-on-a-Chip Suppliers		
Company	Product	Application
Abaxis	Piccolo®, VetScan VS2™	POC (People and Pets)
Affymetrix	GeneChip®	Life Science Research
Agilent Technologies	2100 Bioanalyzer	Life Science Research
Biacore (GE Healthcare)	Biacore Family	Food Quality, Drug Discovery
Biosite Diagnostics	Triage®	POC
Caliper Life Sciences	LabChip®	Life Science Research
Combimatrix	CustomArray™	Life Science Research
i-STAT (GE Healthcare)	i-STAT® Analyzer	POC
Nanogen	NanoChip®	Life Science Research
Sensicore	WaterPOINT	POC (Water Quality)

Source: Bourne Research LLC, 04/07

PART 2

COOL PRODUCTS AVAILABLE TODAY

We live in a society exquisitely dependent on science and technology, in which hardly anyone knows anything about science and technology.

—*Carl Sagan*

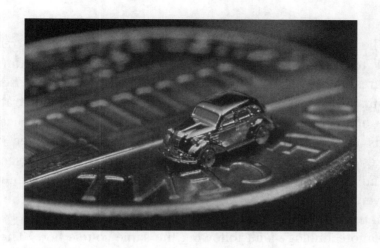

5 • AUTOMOBILES

In 1995, the Guinness Book of Records recognized Nippondenso (now DENSO Corporation) for its creation of the world's smallest car. Using MEMS fabrication techniques, the company's 1/100th replica of Toyota's 1936 Model AA Sedan consisted of 24 individually micromachined parts—including a shell body, chassis, tires, wheels, axles, headlights, tail lights, bumpers, a spare tire and hubcaps. Powered by an electromagnetic stepper motor, it reached a top speed of 10 cm/sec. It is truly a marvel of micro-engineering.

The automobile industry was, and continues to be, an early adopter of MEMS sensors. The first application dates back to 1974, when pressure sensors were tapped to monitor manifold absolute pressure (MAP) in electronic fuel injection systems. Three decades later, and most cars today now rely on about a dozen or so MEMS sensors for a variety of applications. Some high-end luxury vehicles, the BMW 700 Series in particular, utilize several dozen.

The integration of MEMS sensors in cars can be clearly tracked back to one specific use; over the years, their integration has progressively widened, not only across applications, but passenger car makes and models as well. This market clearly illustrates a case of the trickle-down effect. Use for any specific application tends to start in high-end vehicles first, and then, over time, makes their way into cars for the masses. Today, MEMS sensors are an integral part of engine and system management, comfort, convenience and safety, and can be found throughout the car, from the air conditioner to the tires.

Nanotechnology isn't following the same course here. The use of nanomaterials is at its very earliest stages. And there's no one application that is providing the foundation for this growth. Rather, integration is occurring across many different end uses at the same time. The biggest difference with this approach is that fewer models are actually being affected, which may make growth in this sector a little slower than that seen with MEMS. That is, the use won't be as pervasive quite as quickly.

To a certain extent, it could be suggested that MEMS sensors launched the expansion of electronics in cars; or maybe it just happened to take place concurrently. But in either case, manufacturers began to look for an innovative way to monitor power and performance within electronic fuel injection systems. The difficulty was the kind of harsh environment such a sensor needed to withstand—high temperature, oil, etc. A sensor made of silicon seemed ideal for such conditions. Even better, it was small; really small. Once proven, it didn't take long for automotive manufacturers to make use of them for other system functions.

While the integration of pressure sensors proliferated in the 1980s (from manifold absolute pressure to barometric pressure, fuel pressure, oil pressure and more), other MEMS sensors were being developed that would become even more pivotal to the automotive industry. In fact, it's not too far of a stretch by any means to say that MEMS sensors transformed passenger safety when accelerometers found their way into automotive airbags.

Airbags made their debut in the 1970s, when both General Motors and Ford began to explore their use. It wasn't until the late 1980s that manufacturers began to more widely embrace them— primarily due to reduction in cost. Fast-forward roughly 15 years, and airbags have become inexpensive enough that they're not only standard for both the driver and front seat passenger in nearly every car manufactured, but they're also proliferating throughout the passenger compartment.

Today, side curtain airbags are becoming more common, as are those for rear seat passengers. They're also being looked into to protect the legs and feet of drivers, and even pedestrians. Yes, that's right. Some automakers are looking to integrate airbags into the bumpers to better protect those unfortunate enough to be hit by a car. On the surface, that may seem kind of funny, and makes one wonder then if this might make drivers more aggressive around pedestrians, but the fact that such applications can even be considered are a direct result that the use of MEMS accelerometers have had on reducing the price of airbag systems.

But the role of MEMS sensors in safety systems didn't stop with the airbag. In 1996, European automakers began incorporating MEMS gyros from Robert Bosch into cars as part of what they called Electronic Stability Control (ESC), the precursor to today's anti-rollover systems. Because gyros can measure yaw, or rotation, they're an ideal way to make high-performance cars perform even better. Turns can be faster and tighter, since the sensor steps in to make corrections in the event of under- and/or oversteer.

But it quickly became evident that this was a safety system in the making. Now drivers could handle cars better on icy or rainy roads, and loss of driver control was reduced. Coincidentally, ESC quickly became a standard feature in European vehicles at about the same time that consumer groups were highlighting the fact that Sport Utility Vehicles (SUVs), which were selling like crazy in the U.S., had a higher rollover rate than other passenger vehicles, due to their higher center of gravity.

It didn't take long before the U.S. National Highway Traffic Safety Administration (NHTSA) began to conduct a series of internal reviews and safety tests. Their conclusion? In late 2004, NHTSA released a study showing a 35 percent reduction in single vehicle crashes for cars with ESC, and a 67 percent reduction in single vehicle crashes for SUVs with electronic stability control. Two years later, NHTSA announced the mandated inclusion of anti-rollover systems (basically an enhanced version of ESC) in all passenger vehicles, beginning with 2012 models.

What about nanotechnology? It's already playing a role in cars, too. In fact, the first model year to leverage nanotechnology—in the form of a unique seat fabric—was 2000. Nanocomposites made their debut in 2001, followed shortly thereafter by the use of a nanoceramic-based clearcoat (to better protect against fine scratches and swirls). Fuel systems, tires and windshields now all benefit from various nanomaterials, as you will discover in the rest of this chapter. Let's take a look.

Active Suspension

Active suspension (also called dynamic suspension) systems constantly sense changes in the surface of the road and then make any adjustments necessary to improve car performance and responsiveness. As a result, cars with this feature offer superior handling, road feel and even safety. It works via the use of several different components, the most important of which are MEMS accelerometers near each wheel. More advanced systems incorporate hydraulics; in this case, four MEMS pressure sensors are used to monitor hydraulic pressure.

Airbags

In 1984, the U.S. government required that all cars produced after April 1, 1989 include a driver's side airbag. Just four years later, the U.S. National Highway Transportation Safety Administration mandated dual front airbags in all passenger vehicles. Next up and emerging rapidly: side impact airbags.

At the heart of these puffy pillows that can save your life is a MEMS accelerometer, which made their debut in 1991. The sensor measures deceleration, the rate at which a vehicle slows. But, it's been designed to tell the difference between sudden braking and an actual crash.

First-generation airbag designs were found to be lethal to children and smaller women who sit closer to the steering wheel; as a result, second-generation designs deploy at a lesser speed. However, it's critical that passengers are seated at least 10 inches from the bag to avoid injury. This is also where occupant detection systems come in.

Occupant Detection

One of the biggest issues with older airbags was their inability to know anything about the person sitting in the passenger seat. The dangers posed to children, and even small women, are well documented. Airbags deploying too fast for someone sitting too close can be hazardous—even deadly. Today's airbag systems are smarter, thanks to occupant detection technology, which rely on a variety of MEMS devices. The primary benefit is that they ensure that the passenger-side airbag is deployed faster or slower depending on who is occupying that seat.

Today, four different occupant detection systems are in use:

- MEMS strain gauges placed in each corner of the seat bottom to sense relative weight as well as position.
- A silicone-filled balloon (called a bladder) with a MEMS pressure sensor that's placed under the seat cushion.
- A mat comprised of up to 100 MEMS pressure sensors which is embedded into the bottom of the seat to analyze pressure distribution.
- The use of infrared sensors to monitor the entire passenger compartment and determine passenger size, position, etc.

Anti-lock Braking Systems (ABS)

Anti-lock brakes (ABS) are designed to take the challenge out of stopping quickly on wet and/or slippery roads. When a driver hits regular brakes hard, the wheels may lock, causing the vehicle to skid. Wheel lockup can also result in longer stopping distances, loss of steering control, and, if the road is uneven, loss of stability if the vehicle begins to spin. Anti-lock brake systems are designed to sense wheel locking before it occurs and then release the brakes so that locking doesn't happen.

Slipping can occur between the road and the tires without the wheels actually stopping; when this occurs the tires are decelerating rapidly. The system recognizes this through an accelerometer placed on each wheel. When the deceleration of the wheel rises above a certain value, the antilock brake system will engage.

When imminent locking is detected, the antilock system reacts by lessening the hydraulic pressure in the brake cylinders, which disengages the brakes and prevents the wheels from locking. MEMS pressure sensors monitor hydraulic pressure.

Anti-rollover Systems

Electronic stability control (ESC), also commonly referred to as vehicle dynamic control (VDC), is the precursor to anti-rollover technology. Once two slightly separate approaches, they've now been combined into a single system which helps drivers regain control of a vehicle when it starts to skid. They also detect, at an early stage, when a vehicle is about to overturn. The goal is to keep passengers inside the vehicle and to protect them from impact by deploying front and side airbags, as well as seatbelt pretensioners (which tighten the belt) and other safety equipment.

To a certain extent, this system is almost an extension of anti-lock braking by correcting for two situations: oversteer and understeer. ESC systems can better detect spinouts and skidding, and take corrective action. Much like anti-braking systems, the driver may never be aware that the system has intervened. These systems are typically comprised of a MEMS gyro and accelerometer (or two), as well as non-MEMS speed sensors at each wheel.

Batteries

For a five-year period of time, from roughly 1997–2002, the U.S. automotive industry toyed with the idea of producing electric cars, and did so, but in pretty limited volume. The most well-known was General Motor's EV-1. These efforts were due, in part, to several pieces of legislation: the U.S. 1990 Clean Air Act Amendment, the U.S. 1992 Energy Policy Act and regulations issued in 1990 by the California Air Resources Board (CARB) mandating zero emissions vehicles (ZEV). The CARB regulations were later repealed.

Controversy swirls around why these cars were ultimately pulled from the market, with reasons ranging from limited driving range (60–100 miles on a full charge), costs that were too high ($30,000–$40,000 per vehicle) and charge times that were too long (45 minutes to 15 hours). Some claim that CARB repealed ZEV due to pressure from automobile manufacturers, the oil industry and even the U.S. government.

In 2006, interest in electric vehicles again grabbed the attention of the public (and manufacturers), presumably due to all-time highs in gas prices. But things are different this time around. Most important are improvements in design, performance and battery technology. While the first electric vehicle from Tesla Motors is admittedly out of reach of most buyers (at nearly $100k), it's hard to resist a two-seat sports car (and a really cool one at that), that's also environmentally friendly.

The batteries of next-generation electric vehicles are where nanomaterials could make a real difference. In fact, Altair Nanotechnologies sells a lithium-ion battery to power electric vehicles. If that sounds like the same as those involved in the 2006 Dell and Sony laptop battery recall—you're correct. However, using nanoparticles of lithium titanium, rather than graphite, as Altair does with their NanoSafe™ battery, avoids this potentially explosive problem. Even better, their battery provides a driving range of up to about 250 miles on a full charge, and can be recharged in just ten minutes.

The first company to utilize this new battery technology is Phoenix Motorcars in a sport utility truck. However, the truck is being marketed as a fleet vehicle, rather than being available for sale to consumers. The company is targeting government agencies, delivery service firms and even taxis. Trucks with these batteries could be available to the average consumer at some point in the not-too-distant future.

Another nanomaterial-based battery, from A123Systems, currently powers plug-in hybrid electric passenger vehicles that are being evaluated by the South Coast Air Quality Management District for the state of California. Their lithium-ion battery, which benefits from the use of Nanophosphate™ technology, allows such cars to achieve astounding fuel economy—exceeding 150–200 miles per gallon in city driving.

But not just cars are benefiting, and it's not necessarily all about mileage. The KillaCycle, which is said to be the fastest electric motorcycle in the world (going from 0 to 60 miles per hour in less than 1.5 seconds, and driving ¼ mile in just 8.16 seconds), is powered by an A123Systems battery pack.

Finally, did you know about the BMW Hydrogen 7? Said to be one of the first hydrogen-powered luxury vehicles (you can switch between gas and hydrogen with a flick of a switch), the HSS-440 MEMS gas sensor from AppliedSensor is being placed in the passenger cabin, trunk and under the hood to detect for hydrogen, long before such a leak becomes a safety issue.

Body Panels/Trims

As discussed in Chapter 3, nanocomposites offer properties that make a lot of sense for use by automotive manufacturers; and they are indeed slowly finding their way into passenger vehicles. The first known application hit the roads in 2001, when the bumpers of some Toyotas were made of a nanocomposite; their use remains a little hit-or-miss. Examples include:

- 2002 Chevrolet Astro/GMC Safari—optional step assists
- 2005 Honda Acura TL—seat back moldings
- 2004 and 2005 Chevy Impala—body side moldings
- 2005 Hummer H2—trim and panel components of the cargo bed

It doesn't stop there; the diversity really is quite interesting. An interior air vent (found in the Audi A4 and a Volkswagen van) is made of the nanocomposite from Süd-Chemie. Even the mirror housings and door handles of some vehicles are now made of a nanocomposite, and the center console of a 2006 truck is said to be a nanocomposite as well. And they're not all clay-based, although the above examples are. Fenders made of a carbon nano-tube composite can be found on the Renault Clio and Megane.

Cleaning/Detailing

What's the most irritating thing about waxing your car? For me, it's the white residue; although, back in the day when I did actually hand-wax my car, that helped me know which sections weren't sufficiently buffed. In addition, what I dislike about protectant products is that they leave a greasy, almost wet surface wherever it's used, like the dashboard. Well, with the use of nanoparticles, those two issues are a thing of the past. In 2006, two of the leading suppliers of car care products introduced new lines leveraging nanotechnology.

Eagle One is a business unit of Valvoline, a division of Ashland Oil. The use of nanoparticles of carnauba wax in Eagle One's NanoWax® (available in both paste and spray) means that really fine scratches are filled; far better than they are with conventional car wax. As a result, swirl marks are more easily concealed. Even better, there's no white residue. The same goes with their Nano-Polish™ wheel polish, which fills tiny scratches in metal surfaces.

The line also includes the Nano-Protectant™ interior detailer, which provides UV protection of leather and vinyl. This "sun-screen" for your car's interior means your dashboard won't fade as quickly. Even better, the company says that the protectant won't leave a sticky residue.

In the United States, Turtle Wax is a household name when it comes to car care products. In 2006, the company introduced a new line of car care products formulated with nanotechnology, although the company doesn't specifically reveal how. Here's an easy way to check this: if the products have the same properties as those described for Eagle One (the wax dries clear rather than white, and the protectant doesn't leave a wet finish) then it's likely that nanoparticles are in play.

Products include the F21™ Car Wash, F21 Car Polish (available in both a paste and liquid), F21 Spray On Wheel Cleaner, F21 Super Protectant, and the F21 Tire Foam & Shine.

Clearcoat/Paint

It's very possible that the paint of your car is nanoparticle-based, particularly if it has a pearlescent, iridescent, glitter or similar appearance. Chances are it's the Engelhard color effect paint discussed in Chapter 3. Whether the paint is sparkly or not, one concern many car owners have is protecting that paint.

Scratch resistance is a big deal. That's why a lot of buzz quickly generated in late 2002 when word of a nanotechnology-based clearcoat began to get out. Beginning in spring 2004, all E, S, CL, SL and SLK-Class Mercedes rolled off the factory floor with an innovative clearcoat from PPG Industries. Their *CeramiClear*™ product relies on silica (ceramic) nanoparticles, which provide an extremely hard, glass-like surface that increases a car's resistance to fine scratches. It's not available to the general public, but both Mercedes and Nissan now use it when repairing damaged finishes on their respective vehicles.

Climate Control

Too hot? Too cold? Just right? MEMS thermopiles (non-contact temperature sensors) are found in heating control and windscreen de-icing in cars. In this case the sensors read the body temperature of passengers and adjust temperature zones accordingly. Humidity sensors are also slowly finding their way into cars to assist in window de-fogging.

In air conditioners, MEMS sensors monitor compressor pressure. The heart of the AC system is the compressor, a belt driven pump that is fastened to the engine—it is responsible for pumping the refrigerant through the system. When the refrigerant leaves the compressor it's compressed, and therefore has a higher pressure than it had before it entered the compressor. This pressure remains relatively constant until it passes through a metering device where the pressure and temperature are reduced. This low pressure remains fairly constant until it again reaches the compressor and is compressed again.

Tiny MEMS valves are being put to use here too, courtesy of Microstaq, as part of both the pneumatic and hydraulic system. They help control the refrigerant and air passing through the unit.

Displays

Both MEMS and nanotechnology can be found in two new display technologies in cars: heads-up displays and next-generation dashboard instrumentation panels.

Heads-Up Display

The roots of heads-up display (HUD) technology lies with the military, where it was designed to relay data to fighter jet pilots without requiring them to look down at the instrument panel. By projecting vital information, such as airspeed, altitude, and weapons tracking into the pilot's line of sight, while looking out the canopy, reaction times are reduced. As a result, less time is spent rotating the eyes between a possible target and the instrument panel, and more time is focused on the task of hitting the specified military target.

HUD technology was first integrated into passenger cars in the late 1980s, and displayed basic driver information such as speed. HUDs are still offered in a handful of car models (such as the

Chevrolet Corvette) and now display more data, including the speedometer reading, as well as fuel and temperature levels, and are configurable to the driver's data preferences. They currently rely on LCD display technology.

In the very near future are transparent OLED and MEMS-based heads-up displays. Microvision, a leading innovator of optical MEMS technologies, is working with Visteon, a Tier 1 automotive supplier, to bring this market. I've had the chance to give a demo a try and it's pretty cool. While the concept may seem distracting at first, having data such as speed displayed at eye level (on the windshield), rather than looking down at the instrument panel, if only briefly, truly does improve the driving experience.

Instrumentation Panel

A number of cars are replacing LCD displays in the instrumentation panel with organic light emitting displays (OLED). OLEDs are made up of several layers of conductive and emissive materials, resulting in an extremely thin display. The thinnest I've seen so far is about 500 microns thick—with each layer ranging from 100-500 nanometers. They're proving themselves to be much brighter than liquid crystal displays.

Right now, OLEDs are limited to text-based displays that are typically part of what is called the driver information center. As such, they're generally placed in or just under the speedometer. Most of the displays I've seen show one or two lines of text or icons, and are monochrome—although colors include a rich red, blue, green and gold.

One exception is the 2005 Cadillac DeVille STS. It has a one-inch OLED display embedded in the rear view mirror that works in conjunction with two cameras. One provides an image of what's behind you while backing up, and the second allows you to see what's going on in the back seat—which will almost certainly serve to reinforce the fact to young children that mom (or dad) really does have eyes in the back of their head.

Following are some examples of OLEDs in current cars and how they are being put to use:

- Aston Martin DB9—Starting with the 2005 models, two rectangular OLEDs are placed within the speedometer.

- Chevrolet Corvette—Current models include a two-line, blue text display located inside the speedometer; it provides details such as trip computer functions, fuel economy, range and tire pressure.

- Jeep Grand Cherokee—Starting with the 2005 models, there is a small text display of things like what gear the car is in and whether the driver's door is open.

- Mitsubishi Endeavor—This model has one of the most colorful OLED displays to date of various text and icons (in red, blue, green and gold), which shows the speed, whether the bright lights are on and other system functions.

- Toyota Prius—In this car, blue text displays the time, a compass icon, temperature and other functions.

Night Vision

Night vision was first offered in the 2000 Cadillac DeVille. This system employed an infrared sensor that detected heat emitted by objects that may be invisible at night to the human eye. The resulting image was projected as an object in the windshield, in black and white, and in reverse, like a photograph negative. Hot objects, like animals, people, and moving cars, appeared white; cool objects, like trees lining the road, were dark.

Few cars ever made use of the technology, until now. In March 2007, BMW's Night Vision system became available in its 5 Series sedan and wagon, and its 6 Series coupe and convertible. It uses an infrared thermal imaging camera from FLIR Systems, which is based on their MEMS microbolometers.

The Engine

MEMS pressure sensors are used in several ways to monitor engine function, one of which is oil pressure, which is fairly straight-forward. The other two are barometric pressure and manifold absolute pressure.

Barometic Pressure

The barometric pressure sensor (sometimes called a High Altitude Compensator) measures atmospheric pressure, which can vary depending on altitude and even weather. At higher altitudes, the air is less dense, so it has lower pressure; when storms roll in, the atmospheric pressure typically drops. When the car's engine is started, it needs to know what the current atmospheric pressure is so that all of its settings will be relevant to operating conditions at that time. If altitude changes too quickly on the same power cycle, this setting will be in error. This can be one reason why cars seem sluggish while driving up to higher altitudes in mountainous terrain. One way to correct this is to stop and re-start the engine so that it can re-calibrate.

Manifold Absolute Pressure (MAP)

MEMS sensors are used in electronic fuel injection systems to provide information in two areas: mass airflow and manifold absolute pressure. The mass airflow sensor tells the engine about the mass of air entering the engine. This data, combined with information from non-MEMS oxygen sensors, is used to fine-tune the fuel delivery so that the air-to-fuel ratio is just right. The MAP sensor monitors the pressure of the air in the intake manifold. The more air that goes into the engine, the lower the manifold pressure—this reading is used to gauge how much power is being produced by the engine.

A second pressure sensor can also be used here as part of a turbocharged system. Here, air coming into the engine is first pressurized (so that more air/fuel mixture can be squeezed into each cylinder) to increase performance. The turbo sensor operates nearly identically to the MAP sensor, with the difference being that it measures boost (the amount of pressurization).

Oil

Motor oil is an essential component to the car's engine; it helps to cool parts by carrying heat away, as well as to clean and prevent corrosion. It also acts as a lubricant, allowing moving parts to work without causing friction, excessive heat or wear. Over time, tiny microscopic bits of metal are produced from the rubbing of engine parts. The oil filter generally removes these particles, which is one reason why oil needs to be changed.

Interestingly enough, metallic nanoparticles can be added to motor oil to reduce friction and thus extend the life of the engine. A reaction takes place that helps to re-bond and seal the metal. A company by the name of Xado sells a line of synthetic motor oil, engine lubricants and fuel treatments based on their CERMET (ceramic nanoparticles bonded with metal) technology. In 2005, Volvo authorized the use of one of Xado's motor oils under certain conditions; Mercedes Benz followed suit in 2006.

One of the most successful applications of nanofibers to date is in automotive air and oil filters. AMSOIL currently offers the Ea Air Filters and Ea Oil Filters, which rely on a nanofiber instead of the traditional cellulose and/or wet gauze.

Fabrics/Textiles

In 2000, Nissan used the MORPHOTEX® fabric from Teijin for the front seats of its Silvia Convertible Varietta. As described in detail in Chapter 9, it is a really unique fiber that relies on nano-scale layers to reflect light to create color, rather than pigment. To date, I think this is the only car to actually use this material.

Fuel System

Automotive fuel systems, which include the filler neck, inlet check valves, a fuel module (pump/sender unit) inside the tank, the fuel lines and the fuel filter, all have to be designed for electro-static discharge (reducing the risk of static electricity). As a result, these components must be conductive. Since carbon nanotubes are great conductors, fuel line components leveraging such a composite material now include quick connectors, O-rings and the inner barrier layer of filters.

It's hard to say how extensively they're being used; however, one application may give us a hint. The tubing in the flexible portion of the fuel line is also made of a carbon nanotube composite. From Degussa, it's already found in the vast majority of North American cars. (A MEMS sensor is used to monitor the pressure of fuel vapor; it's typically placed on or near the fuel tank.)

Another interesting application of nanotechnology is within the fuel itself. According to Oxonica, when mixed with diesel fuel, their product Envirox™ removes engine deposits and reduces harmful emissions, thus boosting efficiency.

Global Positioning Systems (GPS)

The Global Positioning System (GPS) is a worldwide, radio navigation system comprised of dozens of satellites and their ground stations. The main benefit of having a GPS system in the car is to pinpoint, within a few feet, exactly where the vehicle is.

As a result, the technology continues to gain in popularity, mostly to provide directional guidance (via a display near the dashboard), on how to get to the desired destination, calling for help in the event of an emergency and even tracking the vehicle if it's been stolen.

There are a couple of different approaches in use, ranging from a system fully integrated into the car (such as OnStar), or via the use of a portable GPS system that is taken with you wherever you go, whether you're driving, camping or hiking.

One of the biggest issues with GPS is that signal transmission can be blocked or lost for short periods of time. Obstacles such as mountains, high buildings, tunnels and big trees are the biggest culprits. Even reflections from large surfaces or fences can interfere with the GPS signal.

Leave it to MEMS to come to the rescue (so to speak). MEMS accelerometers help the system stay on track with a dead reckoning approach by monitoring the distance traveled. An even better solution is the more recent introduction of a MEMS magnetic compass, basically a magnetometer (magnetic sensor) with inertial sensing capabilities. In this respect, not only can car movement be monitored, but its direction as well, making the GPS system that much more accurate.

Headlights

Have you noticed some cars have really, really bright bluish headlights? They're not too hard to miss because they're often annoyingly bright. Those are Xenon headlights, a type of High Intensity Discharge (HID) light that first began to appear in the late 1990s. Because of the nature of these lights, keeping them level is of paramount importance. In fact, in Europe, automatic leveling of these headlights is mandatory, as a safety measure, to minimize headlight glare from oncoming vehicles at night. MEMS accelerometers assist in the leveling function.

Tires

Hundreds of millions of tires are manufactured every year. If you have a tire swing, then it's easy to see their structure, which is basically four main pieces: the outermost layer, which is technically called the crown, but most of us simply know it as the tread. The grooves provide traction with the road and are especially useful when it's wet or snowy. The sidewalls are pretty self-explanatory—they are the two sides of the tire. They enclose the inner liner, which is what keeps the air inside. The inside edge of the tire, the one that goes around the rim, is called the bead. There is steel there to help reinforce that edge so it doesn't tear easily.

Today's tires are generally made out of synthetic rubber composites, but some include steel for strength (hence the term "steel belted radial"). The most common filler material used in the composite is silica, or carbon black. So, one could say that tires were probably the first widespread application of nanotechnology, since carbon black has been a tire ingredient for decades. In the past few years, two other nanomaterials have emerged as an alternative: a corn-based nanocomposite and nanoclays.

A tire material co-developed by Goodyear Japan and Novament ranks pretty high on my list of novel approaches. Called Mater-Bi™ it uses nanoparticles of cornstarch to partially replace the more traditional tire filler material silica. If you're in Japan, you'll notice that most Goodyear tires are now marked BioTRED, which means they use this unique material. In Europe, one BioTRED tire is available, the GT3. The use of starch reduces both tire weight and surface resistance, thus improving fuel efficiency.

The Exxpro™ polymer from Exxon, which is currently used as an inner liner for truck tires, relies on nanoclay. The use of nanoclay improves the air barrier in the liner by creating a tight structure that impedes gas diffusion. The result, claims ExxonMobil, is tires that are 20 percent more durable, owing to higher inflation retention and reduction in tire pressure.

In 2004, Yokohama began selling the ADVAN Sport tires, one of the first widely available commercial tires to leverage a nano-composite. The secret recipe is a tread compound comprised of polymer, super-fine silica and an unspecified carbon nanotechnology. According to the company, this gives the tires better grip. Yokohama offers two other lines of tires using its nanocomposite, called S.drive and C.drive.

Also in 2004, ExxonMobil Chemical and Yokohama Rubber announced a joint cooperative agreement and ExxonMobil's acquisition of a global license from Yokohama for their DVA (dynamically vulcanized alloy) inner liner technology. The intent was to develop a new technology based on DVA and Exxpro™. Two years later, in 2006, they revealed its qualification for use in passenger vehicle tires targeted for harsh winter conditions.

A good question is, do tires made with nanomaterials really offer better wear than those made from conventional materials? And if they do, since you won't need to replace them as often, how much more are consumers willing to pay for them?

Tire Pressure Monitoring

In 2000, the widespread failure of Firestone tires, due to separation of the tread, caused more than 270 deaths and 800 injuries in the United States. The fiasco put the spotlight on the use of MEMS pressure sensors, which were just starting to move into the market as a way of monitoring tire pressure.

The highly publicized Firestone/Ford SUV tire recalls subsequently resulted in the enaction of the Transportation Recall Enhancement, Accountability and Documentation (TREAD) Act of 2000. The TREAD Act called for automakers to install tire pressure monitoring systems that warn motorists when tires are dangerously under-inflated, beginning with 2004 models.

Two different technologies are in place. One approach, called the indirect method, relies on a vehicle's antilock braking system, using non-MEMS wheel speed sensors to calculate an estimation of tire pressure. The second, called the direct method, relies on MEMS pressure sensors embedded into the tire itself to monitor tire pressure directly. The direct method is viewed as preferred, given its higher accuracy; as such, it is rapidly becoming the dominant system.

Windshields

Last, but certainly not least, are two products that leverage nanoscale materials to add new life to your car's windshields. NanoFilm sells a product called Clarity Defender™, which basically creates a non-stick surface for the easy removal of things like snow, ice, bugs and dirt.

If regular, boring, colorless windshields aren't your thing, then you'll definitely like a product from PPG Industries, which they call "sunglasses for your car." The blue tint makes your windshield look sort of like a gigantic fly's eye (see the color insert for a photo). But it's not an aftermarket film; rather, it's a nano-composite coating applied during the production process. The most obvious benefit is that it will last longer than a film. Even better, it's more than just good looks. The coating blocks about 90 percent of infrared rays, which helps keep the interior cool.

Vision is the art of seeing what is invisible to others.

—*Jonathon Swift*

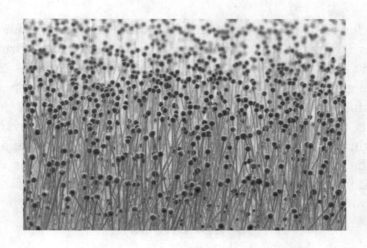

6 • IN AND AROUND THE HOME

When I was kid, I thought for sure that by now we'd be living like the Jetsons, that classic Saturday morning cartoon (when there was still such a thing), set in the fantastic future. A future where we drove to work in a flying saucer, used automatic people movers instead of walking on sidewalks, pushed computer buttons all day, had enormous flat-screen TVs, ate dinners that took just seconds to make and relied on robotic maids. Plus, everything was pristinely clean—from our clothes to our homes.

Wait a minute. Except for the flying saucer part, that almost sounds like how we live today. Many of you probably use a moving sidewalk at the airport, own a huge, flat-screen TV, heat up a pre-made dinner in your microwave and watch as a robotic vacuum cleaner sweeps your floor. To a large extent, MEMS have many of the electronic devices in your home covered.

As for being pristinely clean, well, that's where nanotechnology comes in. Imagine a home where carpets don't stain, furniture doesn't fade, paint doesn't chip and windows are always clean. Nothing looks old, worn or dirty, and all surfaces are germ-free.

If this sounds far-fetched, it's not. Products are already on the market that can do all of the above. They're not widely available though; and some are only for commercial or industrial buildings, not the typical residential home. But the bottom line is clear: MEMS and nanotechnology are making the house of the future a reality today.

Appliances

The appliances that you buy for your home are part of a product category called "white goods." Why? Back in the day, that was the only color available for your refrigerator, stove, washer and dryer. Today's appliances come in all sorts of designer colors; and of course, stainless steel is hot. It's the "it" material of the moment.

In fact, in 2003, AK Coatings, which sells carbon and stainless steel coated with a polymer containing Agion Technologies' silver ions, unveiled a concept home that showcased the extensive use of their product. Some of the home appliance manufacturers that participated were DACOR, Hobart and ICE-O-Matic.

The above is important to point out with more appliances and stainless steel products advertising anti-microbial and/or germ-free properties; but it should be made clear that nanoparticles aren't necessarily being used. That doesn't mean they won't be; it just simply means that, in the case of home appliances, they don't appear to be at this time.

But appliances aren't just the domain of nanomaterials; MEMS sensors are increasingly being integrated to make appliances smarter. One of the most widely used is a thermopile (a non-contact temperature sensor discussed in Chapter 2), but pressure sensors and accelerometers are also increasing in importance.

Cooktop/Stove

Induction cooktops are interesting in that they rely on the use of magnetics, instead of electricity or gas. They're immediately recognizable, since they have a flat, glass-like surface. Coils made of a magnetic material are located just under the surface and cause the pan itself, not the cooktop, to heat up. When the pan is removed, the energy transfer stops. At all times, the cooktop remains, at most, slightly warm to the touch. With an induction cooktop, MEMS thermopiles are used to help regulate temperature by monitoring the temperature of the pan itself.

Have you ever seen (or own) a higher-end gas cooktop in which an exhaust hood comes on automatically when you turn on the burners? If you wonder how that happens, it's actually due to a MEMS thermopile, which senses the temperature change of the cooktop as it starts to heat up.

Dishwasher

In some dishwashers, a MEMS pressure sensor is used as part of the soil-sensing function—it measures the level of soil (food) collected at and passing through the food filter, which then determines the appropriate wash intensity. This is important, because it calculates the amount of water necessary to clean the dishes; thus, this function can be a significant water saver. Other dishwashers use optical sensors instead, which are not as accurate, because they measure how turbid, or dirty, the water is. Something opaque like flour could be misleading in terms of the actual amount of food debris being rinsed off the dishes.

Microwave

The microwave oven has definitely evolved since becoming all the rage in the late 1970s. But did you know that it was actually introduced in 1947? Yet another "accidental" discovery, it was developed by Percy Spencer, a researcher at Raytheon. That first unit weighed some 750 pounds and was 6 feet tall. That's quite a difference from microwaves sold in the 1990s, which could be mounted under the upper cabinets in the kitchen to keep your counter space free.

Today's microwaves are more like ovens, since they're increasingly found installed into the wall just above regular ovens, or combined with convection oven capabilities.

A microwave works by sending microwave radiation through food to cook it; that happens when water absorbs the radiation energy. This is why food with high water content (like frozen food) is better suited to cooking in a microwave than food with a high fat or sugar content. A magnetron is what creates the radiation rays. Despite the power setting you choose, its intensity doesn't change; rather, it turns itself on and off for brief periods of time. These pulses last just seconds. Next time you use your microwave, listen carefully; you can sometimes hear when the magnetron is on and when it's off.

Many microwaves now rely on a MEMS thermopile to monitor the temperature of food as its being cooked to help regulate that brief on/off cycle. In some models, it also allows food to be defrosted and cooked at the same time.

Refrigerator

Ever wonder how refrigerators make ice? It's actually very simple. An ice cube container is automatically filled with water, and when the water is frozen, the cubes are tipped out into the bin. But how does it know when the cubes are ready? In many automatic ice cube makers, a MEMS thermopile remotely detects when the water is frozen.

Speaking of frozen, aerogels could be a really effective insulating material in refrigerators; both in the main unit, as well as the freezer compartment. In fact, nanoskin™ (from General Applications) is now doing just that. The original intent was to apply the technology to portable coolers, like the ones you take on picnics or to your kid's soccer games.

In 2004, Samsung introduced refrigerators with Nano Silver-Seal™, a new application of their Silver Nano Technology. In this case, they created a polymer coating embedded with silver ions. Not only was the inside wall surface of the refrigerator coated with the material, but the filter in the water dispenser as well. The last refrigerator openly advertised to have this coating, the GR-G227STBA, was introduced in April 2006.

Washer/Dryer

With the increased popularity of front loading washing machines, the use of MEMS accelerometers to detect load imbalance is especially important since these machines spin at extremely high speeds. In the past, washing machines used various sensors for this purpose, but none could measure across a wide range of spin speeds. In addition, until recently, MEMS accelerometers were simply too expensive. The price of these sensors is now much lower, so if you have this type of washing machine, a MEMS accelerometer is probably part of it.

During the rinse cycle, rather than filling up with water and agitating clothes, more washers are simply applying a high-pressure spray of water. In this case, MEMS pressure sensors help to regulate water pressure. They're also used to monitor water level in top-loading machines as the tub fills up.

In 2005, Samsung introduced its SilverCare washing machine, which was truly an innovative approach to washing clothes. During the wash and rinse cycles, hundreds of billions of silver ions are released. This allows for the sterilization of clothes without the need for hot water or bleach, but you do still need to use soap.

Given that Samsung's use of silver ions was incorrectly tagged as silver nanoparticles (the company does, after all, refer to it as Silver Nano Technology), they very unfortunately became a poster child of sorts for the growing controversy concerning the use of nanoparticles in general. The ensuing questions raised about possible environmental impact is part of what led the EPA in late 2006 to consider regulating products that advertise anti-microbial properties. As I'm writing this book, the outcome is not yet known.

As for dryers, most simply dry clothes for a pre-determined amount of time. How many times have you discovered that your clothes were still damp after going through your chosen drying cycle? Some dryers use MEMS thermopiles to measure the temperature of clothes so they won't be under- or over-dried. This not only saves energy, but is better for your clothes, since too much heat can be damaging (particularly once they're dry). A few dryers use a MEMS humidity sensor to detect moisture level.

Bed and Bath

In 2006, JCPenney announced that its Studio Brand of 100 percent cotton, 350-count sateen sheets made use of the Coolest Comfort technology from Nano-Tex. What that means is that the fabric draws moisture away from the skin to help keep you cool in the summer and warm in the winter. The same technology is being used in mattresses themselves. The HealthSmart™ mattress from Simmons® not only integrates the Coolest Comfort technology, but Resists Spills as well. The SimplePedic™ luxury mattresses utilize Repels and Releases Stains.

That makes me think about a possible future scenario. Let's say you're enjoying breakfast in bed and you accidentally spill your orange juice (OJ). If your mattress resists spills, and your bedding resists spills, then the OJ would just bead up and roll onto the floor. But then you'd want carpeting (or a wood floor) that uses nanotechnology to resist spills too, so that the carpet won't stain; or at least make it so the wood floor is easier to clean up.

The Bath

A unique approach that many companies are leveraging for cleaning products is what's called the lotus effect. This is because the leaves of the lotus flower are essentially self-cleaning. So when it rains, rather than seeing water spots and bits of dirt left behind, the leaves are clean.

Interestingly enough, this isn't because the leaves are super-smooth, but rather, we now know that they're covered with naturally-occurring nanostructures that are hydrophobic—they repel water. In fact, water droplets on such a surface retain an almost perfectly round shape. As a result, water rolls off, picking up dust and dirt particles along the way.

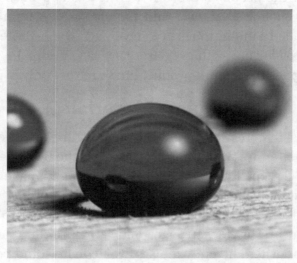

Example of the lotus effect on a treated surface. Photo courtesy of BASF AG.

Degussa offers a surface protection product called Tegotop 105, which combines silica nanoparticles with specialty silicones. When sprayed on a surface, the product creates a layer that repels water. Dirt won't stick either, resulting in the "self-cleaning" effect when the surface is rinsed with water.

A complete opposite approach is making a surface hydrophilic, meaning water can wet it uniformly so it runs off faster. In this respect, water droplets on such a surface are flattened (rather than bead-like), and slide off (rather than roll). Have you ever heard the term "sheeting action" applied to products for use in your dishwasher so that water spots aren't left behind on glassware? This is the same principle. It just works better here because of the nanoscale approach.

A glass cleaner technology called Nano-Protect® (from Henkel) uses silica nanoparticles to do just that. As a result, water drops won't leave marks and the surface stays cleaner longer. However, since the technology makes surfaces attract water, it makes sense that one of the products they offer with this approach is the biff Fresh Shower line of shower and tub cleaners. A family of glass cleaners called Sidolin touch-free leverages Nano-Protect® too—special wipes for use with eyeglasses are also available, which is a fantastic application. Both product lines are sold only in Europe.

Building Materials

Products that resist the effects of moisture and weather the elements better are important properties to the building industry. In this respect, the lotus effect is really starting to make an impact on construction materials and in next-generation insulation. House siding made with nanocomposites are even starting to enter the market that are lighter, stronger and far more durable than the plastic composites currently in use. Even concrete and power tools are now made better in some way with nanomaterials.

Concrete

Southern Clay offers Nanothix® B1490, an additive for cement and gypsum-based products. An example is the mortar used to hold cement blocks together, such as those big bricks that are typically used for foundations. Since it repels water, the result is a joint filler that's more water resistant and less prone to staining.

Sto Corporation sells a product called Lotusan, which is an exterior coating with the self-cleaning effect discussed earlier. It's meant for use on concrete, stucco and fiber cement board, and is available in several dozen colors. I've owned a home with a stucco exterior and have first-hand experience with the fact that dirty stucco is hard to clean—water can make it crack and crumble, and it's also prone to mold and mildew growth; plus, it's a pain to have to re-finish. But I prefer the look of stucco, so I'm all for products that can help it withstand weather better, and stay clean.

Decking

Luxrae recently introduced a line of vinyl composite decking in six different natural-looking wood finishes. Even better, the nanotechnology-based Luxshield coating protects the surface from moisture, stains, scratches and UV rays. Along the same lines, One Time now sells a wood protectant that, when applied, results in a spiky, nanostructured finish. It won't hurt bare feet, but it prevents the spores of mold and mildew from growing.

Insulation

When you think of insulation in your home, I'll bet the first thing you think of is the insulation in your attic and walls. Instead of the traditional pink fiberglass, an interesting alternative is the use of aerogels as a next-generation insulating material. It could be used anywhere conventional insulation is currently found: the roof, exterior walls, the walls of finished basements, and even floors, as well as around windows and doors. Psychologically, it's hard to believe that a material less than an inch thick could insulate better than the 12 to 16 inches of insulation we traditionally use in the U.S., but it's possible.

In the meantime, do you have an insulating blanket on your hot water heater? Have you noticed insulating foam of some sort on the hot water pipes in your basement? If you've bought a home that's fairly old, one of the first things you might notice is that the insulation on those two things are typically old and in not-so-great shape. You might want to consider two innovative approaches made possible by nanotechnology. The first is an insulation blanket made of aerogels.

The second is from Industrial Nanotech, which offers two products for homeowners that are as easy to apply as paint. They provide an easy way to not only add insulation, but moisture control and mold resistance to many surfaces throughout the home as well. In both instances, you apply the product via paint brush, roller or sprayer—just like you would any paint.

Unlike conventional insulation materials, which simply trap air, these products also protect against conduction (this is why the handle of cast-iron frying pan gets hot even though only the bottom is being heated directly), convection (like the heated air draft moving upward from a fire), and radiation (think of the waves of heat from a space heater).

- Nansulate HomeProtect Interior™ is a white coating that is applied to interior walls and ceilings (such as those in attics). It can also be tinted to whatever color you want.

- Nansulate HomeProtect ClearCoat™ is a translucent coating that is applied to all sorts of interior and exterior surfaces—such as HVAC ducts, pipes and water heaters, as well as the walls of basements and crawl spaces. It offers twice the insulating qualities as the interior product.

Going back to the beginning of this section, where I talked about the use of aerogels for wall insulation, Industrial Nanotech recently introduced Nansulate™ Shield, which is basically their insulation material in the form of rolls and sheets, rather than a liquid. They are initially targeting sales to construction firms, but it's only a matter of time before it's available to the consumer.

Tools

If you're going to be a well-rounded contractor and use nano-materials in the building of homes, then you might as benefit from battery-powered tools that rely on nanotechnology.

One of the first batteries to utilize nanomaterials are found in Black & Decker's DEWALT brand of power tools, ranging from a hammerdrill, reciprocating saw and circular saw, to an impact wrench, rotary hammer, jigsaw and flashlight. From A123Systems, the lithium-ion battery utilizes nanophosphate, resulting in a battery that has a lifetime up to 10 times longer with a faster charge time than conventional rechargeable batteries.

Fixtures

Handrails, faucets, door knobs, light switches and the like are all prime candidates for the use of silver to remain germ-free. Right now, Agion Technologies is the leader here with its silver ion approach, but there are a number of companies working to integrate actual nanoparticles of silver in coatings for fixtures such as these, and much more.

Flooring

There's no question that wood floors take a beating. In some respects, a well-aged floor is part of its charm; in other instances, scratches aren't something a homeowner wants to see. If you've installed a wood floor, I'm sure you're aware of the use of some kind of moisture barrier (either in the form of a rubber coating or polymer sheet), but did you ever consider insulating that floor? I sure didn't and wish I'd known about such an option sooner.

Insulation

In late 2006, Industrial Nanotech announced that they were working with Armstrong World, a leading manufacturer of floors, ceilings and cabinets, to incorporate their insulation technology in Armstrong's ceiling and flooring products. So if you buy a drop ceiling, those tiles would have this insulating quality. The concept of floors having insulating properties is really interesting. As a homeowner, you would benefit from insulation and moisture control properties regardless of whether your wood floor or carpet is placed directly on a cement slab or on a wood sub-floor.

Scratch Resistance

BYK-Chemie sells NANOBYK, a nanocoating for scratch resistance using alumina and silica nanoparticles. This isn't a product that consumers can buy, but rather, one that's sold to manufacturers, like those who produce parquet wood flooring.

As for flooring material the consumer can buy, Mirage, a leading manufacturer of pre-finished hardwood floors, uses its Nanolinx™ coating on all of its product lines. Five-times more wear-resistant than conventional coatings, it also has UV protection; depending on the wood, it won't darken or fade.

Furniture

What are the three most important properties to furniture? Stain resistance, fade resistance and scratch resistance. Two days after my new kitchen table was delivered, I put a three-foot scratch in the top. That was five years ago. Today, the likelihood of that happening is greatly diminished, thanks to the development of nanotechnology-based coatings to protect wood furniture.

Two companies currently sell such coatings. These aren't products that consumers can buy, but rather, one that's sold to manufacturers, like those who produce wood furniture. NANOBYK from BYK-Chemie offers both scratch resistance (using alumina and silica nanoparticles) and UV protection (via zinc oxide). EKA (part of Akzo Nobel) sells Bindzil® CC, an additive for clear polymer lacquers used on wood surfaces for improved scratch resistance. It relies on silica nanoparticles.

As for upholstery, the stain resistance technology from Nano-Tex is already being put to use by leading textile firms including Arc-Com, Architex, Carnegie, Designtex, Hunter Douglas Hospitality, Knoll Textiles, Kravet and Mayer Fabrics. What this means is that the fabrics used on chairs and couches will have even greater durability.

If you prefer leather, SolVin, a joint venture between Solvay (a leading producer of vinyl) and BASF, has an interesting alternative. The company recently introduced their first product, NanoVin®, a nanoclay-based composite. One of their target applications is artificial leather within the automotive industry, but I can't imagine that upholstery for furniture, like barstools and chairs, won't be too far behind.

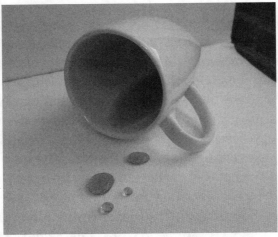

Example of Resists Spills at work. Photo courtesy of Nano-Tex, Inc.

Housewares

The housewares segment is comprised of relatively small items used to cook, like pots and pans, and baking dishes, as well as products that fall under the category of small electrics, like toasters and vacuum cleaners.

There aren't too many examples of nanotechnology being used in housewares, but what's out there is interesting. The same coating that Nanofilm developed for car windshields is also used as a non-stick coating on glass bakeware. Will it give Teflon® a run for its money as a new anti-stick coating for cookware and bakeware? It's a little too soon to tell.

Perhaps the best-known use of silver nanoparticles in housewares is the FresherLonger food containers from The Sharper Image. The integration of silver meant that food wouldn't spoil as fast; that is, it takes longer for the old refrigerator "science project" to come into play. Ok, how many of you have opened up a container only to be faced with fluffy mounds of mold?

Due to the EPA's announcement in late 2006, The Sharper Image no longer advertises the use of silver nanoparticles embedded in the plastic; now they just refer to the containers as being "specially treated."

The instruction sheet that originally came with these containers is a classic example of companies using both "nano" and "micro" to describe the same thing, and often in the same sentence! In this case, the instructions talk about the use of "silver in microscopic particle form," but then point out that the silver nanoparticles average just 25 nanometers in diameter.

Do these containers really work? I haven't given them a try, but those who have say that perishable items with a really short refrigerator life, like strawberries, can be a kept around for a longer period of time—not weeks, but at least several more days—before mold growth sets in.

Toasters

As with older clothes dryers, many toasters simply toast bread based on a pre-determined amount of time. Most of you have probably learned, through trial and error, which setting will result in bread that's toasted to your desired degree of barely golden or nicely charred. Of course, that's just for fresh, sliced bread; never mind figuring out which setting to use for something that's frozen or thicker, like a bagel. If your toaster has some degree of intelligence, it's probably using a MEMS thermopile, which measures the temperature of the bread's surface to determine doneness.

Vacuums

Like many electronics, vacuum cleaners are becoming increasingly intelligent, thanks to the use of various sensors. MEMS pressure sensors help to detect when the bag is full or whether the tube is blocked. It is also used to adjust suction when moving across different floor surfaces, such as from carpet to tile. High-end robotic vacuums that look like the Roomba, but cost thousands of dollars more, use MEMS gyro sensors to help them move around the room and orient themselves.

HVAC

Heating, ventilation and air conditioning (HVAC) systems used in industrial and commercial buildings are increasingly integrating sensors of all kinds (such as MEMS pressure sensors and accelerometers). These automated systems are thus able to monitor and respond to various environmental conditions as a way to reduce energy costs. Automated HVAC is still a rarity in residential homes, but that is expected to change over the next decade.

Beyond sensors, nanomaterials are now starting to play a role here too. The steel for HVAC ductwork, at least that supplied by AK Coatings, now comes with a coating embedded with the silver ions from Agion Technologies for anti-microbial purposes.

The lotus effect is also showing up in a really interesting, but very logical application. Rittal, a leading manufacturer of industrial AC units, recently began using its RiNano coating on their AC heat exchanger coils. Its water, dirt and oil-repellant properties not only keep condenser coils significantly cleaner for a longer period of time, but are also easier to clean. Contamination of these elements can reduce cooling capacity by as much as 50 percent. The product is currently used in industrial environments, but it won't take too long to find its way into consumer HVAC units.

In the meantime, most room air conditioners are moving to the use of MEMS thermopiles to add a much higher degree of intelligence to temperature control. They do so by measuring the surface temperature of objects in the room, as well as detecting things like sunlight shining brightly through the windows, and even the body temperature of people, if present. As a result, it's a much more energy-efficient approach to regulating room temperature.

Lawn and Garden

Many items used in your backyard that rely on plastic or rubber could certainly benefit from a nanoclay-based composite, and some already are, including: fencing, tool sheds, storage containers, the motor casing on riding lawnmowers, even lawn furniture and landscape pipe.

Most patio furniture is now made of either wood or plastic for durability purposes; but in the instance where a lightweight metal is preferred then the Nanoflex™ metal from Sandvik is certainly an option. Since its more corrosion-resistant than aluminum, that makes it especially attractive for outdoor use.

BASF Mincor® TXTT is a self-cleaning coating for tents, awnings, sunshades and other fabrics that you use outdoors. Based on the lotus effect, it makes these textiles hydrophobic so that they're dirt repellant. Of all the things I've seen, this is one of the most appreciated applications of nanotechnology. Outdoor furniture covers are a pain, especially if you like to sit outdoors frequently. It would be nice to go outside and just lightly brush off the cushions, rather than having to beat them to death and still not get all of the dirt out, particularly if you live in a really dusty area like I do.

Several years ago a company by the name of SealGuard USA introduced a line of nanotechnology-based sealants to repel both oil and water-based stains on all types of surfaces, ranging from marble, granite and slate, to brick and concrete. You simply applied it with a paintbrush or roller. It was a great concept for outdoor use in particular, but the company went out of business, so the product is no longer available.

Lighting

Light bulbs are a very interesting application area for nano-materials, with many firms looking for new ways to make light bulbs even more energy efficient. The fact that Australia, Canada and California now propose to eliminate the use of incandescent bulbs (by 2010 for Australia and by 2012 for Canada and California), the need for new light bulb technology is even more important. All three favor compact fluorescent bulbs, but there may be an alternative; and MEMS (of all things) are actually already involved.

Incandescent light bulbs work by passing electric current through a tiny filament wire and heating it; in the process, it creates light. The reason why it's enclosed in glass is because air would quickly oxidize (or basically destroy) the filament. As most of you have probably experienced, this kind of light bulb generates a lot of heat—have you touched one after it's been on? Plus, a 75-watt incandescent bulb lasts, on average, about 750 hours.

Compact fluorescent bulbs (CFL) use 20 percent less energy to produce the same amount of light, and have an average life of 8,000 hours. These properties have made them very popular since their introduction in the 1980s, especially with the elimination of the "flicker" typically associated with early fluorescent lights.

But even CFL bulbs are coming under fire from environmentalists, due to their use of mercury (although we're talking about tiny quantities here). So, there's concern about these bulbs being thrown away and ending up in landfills.

However, there is a third option that most homeowners probably don't even consider—light bulbs based on light emitting diodes (LED) technology. This is probably because these lights are typically associated with intense reds, blues and greens, not the soft white generally desired in home lighting. However, white LEDs as a replacement for incandescent and compact fluorescent bulbs are now becoming available. What really makes them so attractive is their extremely long life; more than 50,000 hours.

The MEMS angle to light bulbs comes courtesy of Celsia Technologies. Their NanoSpreader™ technology, which is a MEMS-based cooling chip, decreases the temperature of LEDs by more than 50 percent. They aren't particularly hot to begin with, but this heat reduction does help to extend life.

The Lighting Science Group, a leading producer of LED light bulbs, is using the NanoSpreader™ in their ODL® Low Bay lighting fixtures (for commercial applications) and LED R30 light bulbs for consumers. Along the same lines, Chip Hope, a leading producer of LED-based street lights, is also using the cooling technology. The end result is street lights that use less energy, last longer, and offer a better quality light.

Paint

Paint—whether it's for the inside or outside of your house— seems like a natural application for nanoscale ingredients, especially pigments, or what gives paint its color. But that's just a start, as you're about to see.

Interior Paint

In 2006, BEHR Paints introduced the first known paint of its kind to leverage nanoparticles. Because of this, BEHR Premium Plus Interior Sateen Kitchen and Bath Enamel dries with an extremely hard, durable finish. That makes it more water resistant, decreasing the chance of mildew growth—the surface is also less prone to stains and easier to wash. You might think that a harder finish would make it more likely to chip, but actually, the opposite is true; it's less prone to chipping.

Exterior Paint

BASF sells a product called COL.9® which was specifically developed for use in exterior coatings and paints. It's a binder comprised of inorganic nanoparticles in a polymer; the result is resistance to dirt and cracking, so paint will last longer. Even more interesting is the fact that it doesn't melt during fire. I never considered that as a firefighting hazard, but it makes a lot of sense. In fact, "no melt no drip" is a requirement for many military technologies, particularly those that are metal or fabric-based.

One of the first known product lines based on COL.9 is Herbol-Symbiotec™ from Akzo Nobel. The Herbol® brand of professional architectural paints and coatings became available in early 2007. They're extremely dirt repellent, and don't fade as quickly as conventional products. Celanese Corporation sells a similar product called Mowilth® Nano, which forms a nanostructured surface for increased durability.

Lead Paint Concerns

More than three-quarters of homes built in the U.S. before 1978 contain lead-based paint; the same holds true for most commercial and industrial facilities. Removal and replacement of that paint can be very expensive—more than a trillion dollars have been spent on such efforts in the U.S. alone.

Industrial Nanotech has an alternative that costs far less. Their product, Nansulate LDX is a clear, industrial coating that encapsulates lead painted surfaces. Two coats applied to the surface in question apparently form a long-lasting seal that removes the danger of the lead paint.

Windows

Windows are a very important component to homes; in some ways, they give the house its character. Beyond architectural significance, windows can be a major source of energy loss; they can also be a pain to clean. How much do you like washing windows? The use of nanoscale materials is allowing manufacturers to develop windows that are "smart" in a number of ways.

Heat Reduction

3M has a new line of window films, called the Prestige Series, which offers a number of interesting features. The most intriguing is that nanomaterials eliminate the need for metal in the film, which the company says can interfere with cell phone signals. Plus, the use of nanoscale materials in the creation of this film offers the kind of features that we now know they can provide. This film not only reduces the amount of heat coming through the window and blocks UV rays to slow fading, but reflectivity is also reduced, so it won't seem like you're looking through a film.

While window films are a do-it-yourself project for home-owners, an alternative is for manufacturers to use new insulating materials in the manufacture of windows themselves.

For example, Cabot Aerogel and Wasco Products created a sky-light (for commercial use) incorporating aerogel. Available via Wasco, the Thermalized® Solar-Energy Skydome® system, with Nanogel®-filled polycarbonate panels, offers more than double the thermal performance of standard skylights, while minimizing glare and heat gain. They also resist condensation, reducing the growth of mold and mildew. Another line of skylights leveraging Cabot's aerogels are available from a company called ACRALIGHT International Skylights.

Cabot's Nanogel® is also found in windows by Kalwall, Super Sky Products, Westcrowns, Scobalit, GE Advanced Materials Structured Products, Okalux and Pilkington. But Pilkington's glass is actually better known for its self-cleaning properties.

Self-Cleaning

Pilkington Activ™ Self-Cleaning Glass relies on a coating that reacts with sunlight to break down dirt (called a catalytic effect). Plus, because the glass is hydrophilic (meaning water doesn't bead), it runs off the glass in a sheet—much like when you spray water on a window. And the dirt goes with it. So, after it rains, rather than having a dirty window (because of the water spots and subsequent dirt left behind), the windows are actually cleaner. How cool is that?

The company prefers to refer to their product as a thin-film technology, which indeed it is. But the fact that this film of titanium dioxide is just 15 nanometers thick, it does fit within the scope of nanotechnology. At the micro scale, this product just wouldn't be possible.

A similar product is available from PPG Industries. Their Sun-clean® Glass is for residential window applications and uses the same photocatalytic properties in its coating to break down dirt. This thin film (which contains nano-particles) also sheets water so that rain, or even the spray from a garden hose, cleans the windows. Actually, back in 1983, PPG introduced a low-emissivity glass, Sungate™ 100, in which a nano-thin layer of material filters out infrared radiation from the sun and keeps heat inside.

If self-cleaning windows aren't part of your remodeling plans, you could use a window cleaner that provides the same, if only temporary, effect. Eurochem Chemical now sells Clear View 66, a combination glass cleaner and sealant that helps to protect against bird droppings, acid rain, color fading and general pollutants. It's targeted to the professional window cleaning industry, but it makes sense that homeowners will be next.

So, what do you frame these great self-cleaning windows with? Well, curtains of course. And what better than those from Komatsu Seiren (which they developed in conjunction with Toray Industries). They have a unique nanostructure, which means that grains of pollen won't stick to them. Yes—they're anti-pollen.

Normal people...believe that if it ain't broke, don't fix it. Engineers believe that if it ain't broke, it doesn't have enough features yet.

—*Scott Adams (creator of the Dilbert comic strip)*

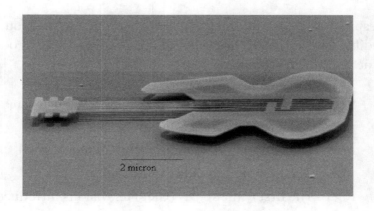

2 micron

7 • CONSUMER ELECTRONICS

With cell phones, video games and MP3 players such an integral part of our lives, it's hard to believe that we ever communicated or entertained ourselves without them. Looking back just twenty years, the concept of rotary phones, an electronic game called "Pong," and playing a stack of single-song 45's on your stereo turntable seem almost quaint in comparison. However, while the electronic devices of today are modern conveniences, their technological roots are actually quite ancient.

The basic principle of optics was known to both the Chinese and the Greeks in the 5th and 4th centuries BC—three thousand years ago. As we now know, optics technology is an important component in many of today's consumer electronic products, from digital TV and DVD players, to the communications infrastructure that supports the Internet. Let's take a quick look at how far we've come in a relatively short period of time, focusing on some of the key "firsts" in the evolution of consumer electronics.

Despite being such an integral part of our daily lives, I found it incredibly interesting to learn how long some of these products have actually been around.

- 1826—The first photographic image taken with a camera
- 1888—The first mass-market camera
- 1910—The first talking motion picture demonstrated
- 1920—The first ready-made radios sold
- 1934—The first cathode-ray (CRT) televisions introduced
- 1951—The first computers sold commercially
- 1962—The first computer game invented
- 1964—The first computer mouse demonstrated
- 1969—The introduction of ARPANET (the foundation of the Internet)
- 1972—The first home video game consoles sold
- 1977—The first cell phones demonstrated
- 1979—The first portable audio player introduced
- 1980—The first portable camcorder demonstrated
- 1981—The first laptop computers sold
- 1984—The first digital camera demonstrated
- 1994—The World Wide Web is born

Cell Phones

The 1990 movie "Pretty Woman" provides a great visual example of how far cell phones have come in such a relatively short amount of time. In an opening scene, you see a businessman walking down the street talking on the latest, greatest gadget: a cell phone. The handset is about the size of a 16 oz. bottle of soda and attached (by a cord no less!) to a battery back, which is worn over the shoulder like a messenger bag. The image is funny considering that today's cell phones are the size of a small candy bar (battery included). And all you could do back then was talk to people.

Fast-forward two decades and today's cell phones are rapidly becoming less phone-like and more like portable, multi-functional entertainment consoles: you can talk, text-message, email, take pictures, capture video, play games, listen to music, watch TV and much, much more. And a lot of this functionality is coming courtesy of MEMS. Really.

Avago Technologies got things rolling about five years ago with an RF MEMS device called the FBAR duplexer. They've since expanded to filters and front-end modules. As I explained in Chapter 2, these components help cell phones work more efficiently as they switch between different cell phone bands and internal functions. More recently, MEMS microphones made their move into cell phones as a higher-quality replacement to the condenser electret microphones currently used.

But what's really making news is the integration of MEMS accelerometers. Annual production of cell phones now exceeds one billion, with hundreds of new models introduced each year. These sensors have found their way into less than two dozen models over the past few years, but the way they're being put to use is quite interesting.

Here's a historical timeline of MEMS accelerometers in cell phones to date and the features they're allowing handset manufacturers to offer:

- July 2003—MyOrigo's MyDevice demonstrates the use of a dual-axis accelerometer for screen orientation (to rotate between a horizontal and vertical position depending on how you use the phone).

- September 2003—NTT DoCoMo's RAKU RAKU III phone also functions as a pedometer.
- May 2004—Nokia's 3220 has a clip-on frame (called the Xpress-On™ Fun Shell) that you wave to create short messages. It's "air texting" at its best.

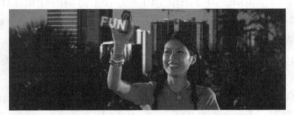

How the Xpress-On Fun Shell works. Photo courtesy of Nokia.

- June 2004—Vodaphone's V4011D offers screen orientation, works as a pedometer, and has gaming control (you tilt and shake the phone to play the game).
- January 2005—Samsung's SCH-S310 is completely keyless; you simply wave it in the shape of the numbers you want to dial.

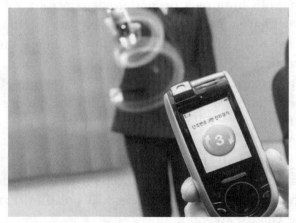

Dialing without a keypad. Photo courtesy of Samsung Electronics.

- January 2005—Pantech's Curitel PH-S6500 is one of the first with both a tri-axis accelerometer and a tri-axis magnetic sensor to function as a pedometer and for gaming control.

- February 2005—Vodaphone's V603SH offers screen orientation and gaming control.

- June 2005—LG's SV360 and KV3600 use an accelerometer for gaming control.

- October 2005—Samsung's SGH-E760 relies on an accelerometer to launch and interact with programs (you shake the phone to skip MP3 tracks or adjust volume) and for gaming control.

- February 2006—Vodaphone's 904SH offers a GPS map (the accelerometer adjusts the map on the screen according to the direction you're facing) and the ability to identify star constellations depending on where you point the phone in the sky.

- May 2006—Nokia's 5500 Sport Phone relies on a tri-axis accelerometer to function as a pedometer.

- May 2006—Sony Ericsson's W710 Walkman® phone works as a pedometer.

- January 2007—Apple's iPhone relies on a tri-axis accelerometer to rotate the display between portrait and landscape mode.

- January 2007—KTFT's EVER 360 (EV-KD370) uses an accelerometer for screen orientation (an important feature since this phone offers mobile TV) and to change MP3 tracks by shaking the phone.

- March 2007—Sony Ericsson's Z750 and W580 also function as pedometers.

But accelerometers aren't the only MEMS device to offer unique features. In late 2005, LG Electronics introduced a line of three phones (the LG-SD410, LG-KP4100, and LG-LP4100), which also functioned as a breathalyzer, using a gas sensor to detect alcohol by sensing traces of ethanol.

For the most part, the majority of the above phones are only available in either Japan or South Korea. A few were launched in Europe and a couple of models are sold in the United States.

As for nanotechnology, that's coming into the play as well—sort of. In late 2006, Motorola announced the launch of the i870 phone with an anti-microbial coating, courtesy of Agion Technologies. However, Motorola incorrectly describes the use of zeolites as nanoparticles, which caused some confusion at the time.

The real nanotechnology angle in some cell phones today is the use of OLEDs—organic light emitting displays. The basic structure of this technology reminds me of an open-face sandwich, with several layers of different materials.

On the bottom is a substrate, which is typically made of clear plastic or glass. On top of that is an anode, which removes electrons when current flows through it. Next are two layers of organic compounds. One is a conductive layer (made from organic plastic molecules) and the other is an emissive layer, which is what emits the light. The final layer is a cathode, which injects electrons when current flows through it. The movement of electrons through these layers is basically what creates light. The entire structure is just 100 to 500 nanometers thick.

OLED displays are brighter and use less power than liquid crystal displays, which is why they're making their way into consumer electronics such as mobile phones, digital audio players, portable media players and even watches. Right now, they're mostly used as a way to display a few lines of monochrome text or simple graphics (in a rich blue, green, red or gold). If you have a newer clamshell (flip) phone with an external display, that may be nanotechnology (in the form of an OLED display), right in the palm of your hand.

Full-color displays are indeed available, but hard to find; it may be because they're very difficult to view in sunlight. Only a handful of cell phone models use OLEDs as the main display—known phones include Haier's Black Pearl, Nokia's 6215i and several from Philips' Xenium line. Other examples include the ZEN Micro-Photo, ZEN V, and ZEN Plus from Creative, but those are digital audio players.

Who makes OLED displays? Samsung, Kodak and Cambridge Display Technology are some of the leading manufacturers.

Digital Cameras/Camcorders

In keeping with our discussion about OLED displays, the technology made its move into digital cameras several years ago, when Kodak introduced the EasyShare LS633. The camera had a 2.2-inch full-color, OLED display, but I haven't seen anything since, with the exception of Sanyo's Xacti HD1 Digital Media Camera, a camcorder. The technology is out there, it's just not widely used right now. In the meantime, MEMS inertial sensors are making their way into digital cameras and camcorders, for image orientation and stabilization.

Image Orientation/Stabilization

Just as accelerometers re-orient the screen of a cell phone from portrait (vertical) to landscape (horizontal) mode, depending on how you're holding it, the sensor is being put to use in digital cameras to detect whether the camera is being held horizontally or vertically while taking a photo. That way, once you download the image, you don't have to spend the time to re-position it so you can view or print it easily. Canon is at the forefront here with their Intelligent Orientation Sensor; many of their PowerShot digital cameras now have this feature.

One of the biggest issues with camcorders when they first hit the market was hand jitter; the noticeable (or not so noticeable) movement of one's hand when holding the camcorder while filming resulted in blurry video. As a result, optical image stabilization (OIS) was born. It's primarily a software algorithm to compensate for shaky hands; however, the recent addition of a gyro sensor (or two) is making these systems even better. They correct for a wide range of camcorder motion, ranging from the obvious, such as vibration while filming in an airplane and hand tremble, to the not-so-obvious, such as body sway (even if you think you're standing perfectly still). The end result is crisp video images.

Gyro-based optical image stabilization isn't found in all camcorders, but two systems are known to use them: Canon's *Super-Range* OIS and Sony's Super Steady Shot® OIS. In early 2007, Sanyo introduced the Xacti CG6 series, which uses a gyro sensor to detect and compensate for camera shake.

Computers

In 2003, IBM introduced two new ThinkPad® models (the R50 and T41) with an intriguing new feature: an Active Protection System. What it does is protect your computer, should you accidentally drop it or it falls off the desk onto the floor, by preventing the hard drive from crashing.

A computer's hard drive looks a little bit like a record player. The record part is called the platter, which is where data is recorded. At the tip of the arm is the read/write head, which does just that: read and write data on the platter. When not in use, the arm (and head) swings over to the side and parks, so that it's no longer over the platter.

If you drop your computer while data is being read or recorded, there's a high probability of damage. With the Active Protection System, if the accelerometer senses free-fall (or zero gravitational force), it sends a signal for the hard drive to swing the head away from the platter and park it, keeping your data safe.

Apple followed suit in 2005, when they launched the new PowerBook® G4, which featured their Sudden Motion Sensor technology. Also referred to as a Mobile Motion Module, the system is now found in many new Apple computers.

Where this technology is mostly being put to use is in micro-drives, particularly those from Hitachi and Seagate Technologies. If you have a cell phone with a microdrive, chances are pretty good that it has drop protection. That makes a lot sense since people seem to be more prone to dropping their cell phone than their laptop computer.

Another MEMS device moving into computers is the silicon microphone. Fujitsu's LifeBook® T4215 convertible Tablet PC uses microphones from Akustica. Why does a microphone matter in a computer? Well, most don't have them to start with. If you make phones calls over the Internet, one of the first things you probably needed to do was buy an external microphone to plug in (at least before VOIP phones became available).

As for nanotechnology, LG Electronics coated the cooling fan in the TX EXPRESS with carbon nanotubes in order to decrease heat. Next time the fan on your computer is running, hold your hand over the vent. The air that comes out is pretty hot. Reducing this heat can help increase your computer's efficiency.

Printer Paper

I talked about the use of MEMS in ink jet printing at length in Chapter 2. Yet there's another angle to touch on: paper. Nanotechnology actually plays a much bigger role in paper production than many realize—and I'll discuss this in more detail in Chapter 12. But it makes sense to mention a new line of paper here, since it's targeted for use with digital cameras.

If you're like many who have a color ink jet printer to print out photos, you might want to consider Kodak's Ultima Photo Paper with COLORLAST technology. It's comprised of nine layers of ceramic nanoparticles and other coating materials that make it far more resistant to heat, humidity, light and ozone; that means they won't fade nearly as fast. According to the company, photos printed on this paper will last for more than 100 years when displayed under normal conditions in the home.

Gaming

In 1989, Nintendo introduced a portable, handheld gaming console called the Game Boy, which quickly became one of the most popular video game systems developed. More than a decade later, in early 2001, Nintendo extended their popular Kirby video game series by introducing Kirby Tilt 'n' Tumble. As far as I know, it was the first, and remains the only, known game to have a MEMS accelerometer sensor built right inside the cartridge itself, making it an integral part of game play. As with many video games, there are multiple levels, each laid out where you must roll Kirby (a little puffball) through a series of mazes comprised of platforms, bumpers, holes, conveyor belts and more—in this case by tilting and shaking it.

Sound familiar? It should if you own the Nintendo Wii™. In late 2006, Nintendo changed video gaming as we know it with the introduction of the Wii. What makes the system so unique is that Nintendo completely re-designed the game controllers to leverage the use of tri-axis accelerometers. It was, in a word, revolutionary.

Over the years, game players became used to a wing-like controller which they hold with both hands. No more. The main controller of the Nintendo Wii looks like a simplified television remote, and has a tri-axis accelerometer from Analog Devices embedded inside. The secondary unit, the Nunchuk™, benefits from a tri-axis accelerometer from STMicroelectronics.

Suddenly, playing video games is no longer an individual, passive activity. The controllers allow you to get up off your butt and participate. It didn't take long before blogs started mentioning how people were losing weight while playing with the system.

Even better, the Wii seems to be a catalyst for socialization—amongst families, neighbors and even nursing home residents. Now you can easily organize a bowling league or tennis match, and you don't have to go any further than your own living room. Well, maybe down the street to your neighbor's house.

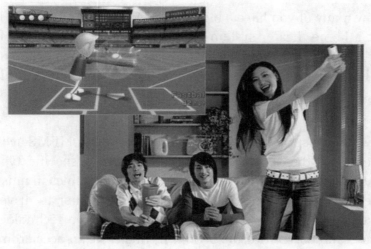

Playing baseball in your living room. Images courtesy of Nintendo.

Until the Nintendo Wii, the use of accelerometers in video game systems was pretty much hit or miss. A number of controllers, including a few joysticks and some unique peripherals (such as snowboards), gave it a try, but they didn't do particularly well.

Sony's new SIXAXIS™ controller for the PLAYSTATION®3 relies on inertial sensors for six-degrees-of-freedom sensing, but in the conventional wing design.

A video game that leverages a tri-axis accelerometer (this time from Freescale Semiconductor) is generating a lot of good buzz: Guitar Hero II™ from RedOctane®. Introduced in late 2006, the game controller is a not-quite-full-sized electric guitar. Instead of strings, you push buttons to play chords. Once you get the hang of it, it's addicting. Basically, flashing lights show you which chords to play so you can replicate a pretty good cover list of known rock songs; the better you play, the louder the crowd screams their approval. You really do feel like a rock star.

Home Theater/TVs

How many of you have a big-screen TV? Surround sound? How about a home theater system? If you answered yes to any of the above, chances are a few MEMS devices are working hard to make your home entertainment experience as rich in sound and vision as possible.

Audio

If you have surround sound, it's possible that a MEMS accelerometer is in the subwoofer. Subwoofers are a specific type of speaker used to reproduce the low booms and rumbles in music or movies. Active subwoofers have a built-in amplifier to drive the speaker (creating the sound), and many use servo technology to measure and correct for distortion. In this case, an accelerometer is part of the speaker driver's diaphragm to measure the movement of the driver. If it does not match the ideal movement (or input signal), then it's adjusted on its way to the amplifier. This results in the most distortion-free sound available. A few of the companies who use this approach include Bang & Olufsen, Genesis Advanced Technology and Velodyne.

Home Theater Projectors

Home theater was once the realm of the wealthy few. You needed enough space to set aside for couches or theater seating, not to mention a screen and the installation of a large, heavy, very expensive projector. That all changed in the late 1990s.

Even as Texas Instruments' DLP® was transforming the business projector market (making them truly portable for traveling), the technology began finding its way into home theater. With the concurrent explosion in DVDs, the timing couldn't be better. Suddenly, it was possible to watch a movie at home with the same kind of quality you'd see in a movie theater.

Today, home theater is a reality for the masses. Forget the need for a special room in the house, and spending hundreds of thousands of dollars. Today's systems cost just a fraction of that and are portable. You can set up your home theater when you want, where you want. And it's not just for movies (although I heard great stories early on of people projecting movies on the back wall of the house during the summer and watching while floating in the pool). Enjoy the super bowl on your living room wall or play your favorite video game on a room-size display. How's that for taking the Nintendo Wii to a whole new level?

Televisions

First, liquid crystal displays (LCD) shook things up as a replacement for CRT (cathode-ray) TVs. Then it was plasma's turn; suddenly, TVs were flat enough to hang on a wall like art. For a brief moment, in early 2006, the electronics world toyed with the thought of a TV display based on carbon nanotubes (until a lawsuit basically put an end to that). Now, OLEDs are being touted as the next big thing for your living room. Don't hold your breath for a big-screen version anytime soon though; the largest demonstrated prototypes at this point are less than 30 inches.

Through it all, Texas Instruments' DLP® quietly found its way into the market. Most probably don't know this, but DLP is giving plasma a real run for its money. Today, you have your choice of more than 75 television models leveraging tiny MEMS mirrors. Samsung is a real leader here, and their newest model, the HL-S4676S, is just 10.6" deep. Even better, this 46" TV is a feather-weight at just 46.3 pounds; nearly *half* the weight of a 46" plasma TV, which weighs in at 83 pounds.

A next-generation alternative to your complicated, button-laden television remote comes courtesy of Hillcrest Labs. The Loop™ is a donut-shaped controller with two buttons and a scroll wheel, and uses their Freespace™ motion control technology to control the device. MEMS inertial sensors allow you to navigate through on-screen menus, then point and click. However, The Loop™ is part of Hillcrest Labs' HōME™ Interactive Media System (which is sold as part of a cable system), so unfortunately, it's not available as a stand-alone universal remote.

Toys

Do you remember Sony's AIBO (Artificial Intelligence based ROBOT)? The cute little robotic dog sold out in something like 15 minutes when introduced in 1999, despite a steep price tag of $2500. The crowds were unreal when the company demonstrated it at the Consumer Electronics Show; it was the most incredible thing we (pretty much everyone there) had ever seen. AIBO was one of the first toys to benefit from the use of a MEMS sensor. In this case, an accelerometer, which helped AIBO sense whether someone picked it up or if it fell over.

Just two years later, Omron followed with NeCoRo (nicknamed Max). Few people outside of Japan know about the toy, but it takes AIBO a step further by encasing it in plush, just like a stuffed animal. The cat will purr, turn its head, move its ears, blink its eyes, and can sit or lay down. Like, AIBO, it relies on an accelerometer for orientation. It costs roughly $1300.

For the next few years, both Sony and Honda worked on creating more advanced robots, in the form of Qrio and ASIMO, respectively. These bi-pedal robots, which stand on two legs, just like a person, can not only walk, but dance and stand up by themselves if they fall, thanks to the use of gyro sensors and accelerometers. Although not available as commercial products (and certainly not as toys), they showcased the range of abilities that such sensors provided.

The newest iteration of robotic toys, in the same vein as Qrio and ASIMO, is PLEN the Desktop Hobby Robot from Akazawa Japan. Just nine inches tall, this bi-pedal robot has 18 moveable joints. A tri-axis accelerometer allows it to dance and stand up if it falls down; it even does a karate kick and can ride a skateboard.

The robot is most impressive when roller skating. PLEN can balance on one foot as it bends over with outstretched arms and one leg up in the air, or stand upright, with its arms behind its back, re-creating the movements of an in-line skater out for a leisurely Sunday roll around the park. As with AIBO and Max, it's not inexpensive. The company made only 50 (priced at $2399 each), although they may make more if there's enough demand.

A less expensive version comes courtesy of TOMY. The i-SOBOT is just 6.6-inches tall and can also walk, dance and do karate kicks—thanks to a MEMS gyro—for just $350.

One thing that's important to point out here is that, while there are a lot of toys on the market with sensors (some of the most sophisticated being Pleo from Ugobe, and the robotic pony from Hasbro), these don't necessarily use MEMS sensors just yet. A good indicator is price, and that threshold now seems to be around $300. If it's more than that, the chances are pretty good that a MEMS sensor of some sort is in play. If it's less than that there probably isn't; at least right now.

Nanotechnology is finding its way into toys as well. In early 2007, Pure Plushy introduced a line of stuffed animals by the same name. These particular toys are filled with memory foam (a super-soft foam that bounces back to its original shape after being compressed), which is infused with silver nanoparticles to keep it germ-free. This internal approach is an interesting alternative to the use of silver ions or nanoparticles on the exterior of such a toy.

More Cool Stuff

The concept of wearable displays had been around for many years; they were originally designed for use with laptops for mobile computing. But, beyond being an interesting idea, they've never been commercially successful. One big reason was the geek factor; they weren't "cool" looking. Never mind the fact that many early headsets completely blocked off your peripheral vision, resulting in claustrophobia and even nausea. Not anymore.

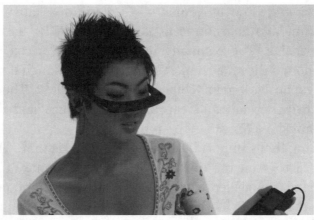

A wearable display you can take anywhere. Photo courtesy of myvu Corporation.

One wearable display that could change things is the myvu® which relies on the use of a tiny MEMS mirror to project an image. Not only that, but it's kind of cool looking (in a retro 1980s sort of way), and allows you to see what's going on around you. In a testament to how times change, they're currently designed for use with Apple's iPod®; those that play video, of course.

In early 2001, buzz began to swirl around a secret project involving inventor Dean Kamen; something that was going to transform our lives. Referred to as both "Ginger" and "IT", speculation ran rampant. Was it a new form of energy? Was it a space-age transport system? Whatever it was, it would revolutionize the world. Over the course of 9 months, the hype grew to near-frenzy levels. When the Segway® Personal Transporter (PT) was finally revealed in late 2001, the disappointment was clear. Many simply thought, 'oh, it's a *scooter'*.

Not even close. I thought it was unbelievably cool; but then, I knew the reason why the Segway PT worked the way it did: MEMS sensors. What tipped me off was Dean Kamen's work on another product that I was keeping a very close eye on: the INDEPEN-DENCE® iBOT® Mobility System (see Chapter 11).

At the core of the Segway Smart Motion™ technology is a cluster of MEMS gyro sensors and accelerometers; what they do is provide balance, just like when you're walking. Stand up straight; take a step forward, and what happens? You remain upright, or at least you should. The same thing happens as you walk and turn left; you've changed direction, but you remain upright. Even standing still, your body's sense of balance keeps you upright as you lean forward and backward, or to the left and right.

The inertial sensors detect these shifts in movement and then make the necessary adjustments to maintain balance. So, if you lean forward, you'll move forward. If you lean to the right, you'll turn to the right. When you stand up straight, you'll stop. The end result is something that mimics human balance while walking; except, rather than using your legs, you glide on two wheels. Once you get used to it (which takes just a few minutes), it's absolutely effortless, and an awful lot of fun.

The Segway i2 is ideal for commuting or just rolling around town; they're also used by police departments, in warehouses, at theme parks and even on cruises. The Segway x2 is a new "off-road" model with more rugged wheels for use while playing golf or simply having fun on dirt trails.

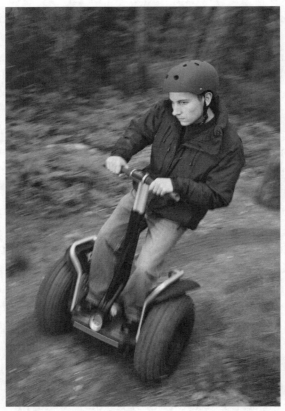

Off-roading fun with the Segway x2. Photo courtesy of Segway Inc.

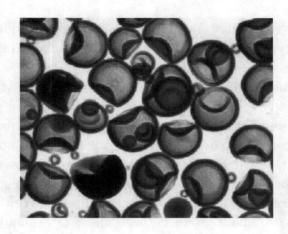

8 • PERSONAL CARE

What's in your medicine cabinet? Chances are there's a fairly extensive assortment of make-up, skin care, fragrances, toiletries, hair care products, sun care products, razors, shaving cream, deodorant and soap.

Personal care is a multi-billion dollar business, with cosmetics generating more than $255 billion globally in 2006. The top ten beauty and personal care companies alone accounted for more than a third of total revenues, and eight of these firms are known to have products which leverage nanoscale ingredients in some form or another.

There's a lot of controversy about this. The key issues are how deeply can nanoparticles penetrate the skin, whether they can enter the bloodstream, and if so, then what? These are absolutely legitimate questions. But this book isn't the appropriate place to make the case that nanoparticles are (or aren't) safe. I don't want to appear as though I'm glossing over the matter, but there are others more qualified than I who can better address these concerns. My intention with this chapter is to help you make sense of what is, essentially, a minefield of industry jargon.

The cosmetic industry has long come under fire for using a lot of big words to sell what many believe to be nothing more than "useless potions" at a premium price. But it's not all propaganda; these companies employ thousands of scientists and spent nearly $1 billion on research and development in 2006. However, with the science behind cosmetics becoming more sophisticated, beauty firms are straddling an increasingly thin line between marketing hype and claims about products that some believe should result in their being classified as drugs.

According to Section 201(I)(1) of the U.S. Federal Food, Drug, and Cosmetic Act, cosmetics are "articles intended to be applied to the human body for cleansing, beautifying, promoting attractiveness, or altering the appearance without affecting the body's structure or functions." This includes products such as skin creams and lotions, perfume, lipstick, fingernail polish, eye and facial make-up, shampoo, hair color, toothpaste and deodorant, as well as "any ingredient intended for use as a component of a cosmetic product."

The key point here is that these products are not allowed to affect the body's structure or functions. If they do, they must be regulated as a drug. Adding nanotechnology to the mix is only serving to complicate matters. For one thing, using ingredients at the nanoscale allows them to penetrate deeper into the skin to visibly improve its appearance. Some believe that crosses the line in terms of function. Others are more concerned about whether the use of nanoparticles is harmful.

Given the growing controversy, in late 2006, many beauty firms removed all reference to "nano" from their websites and marketing materials. And with the amount of money involved, there's a lot at stake. However, what's interesting is that most of the ingredients currently used fall within the spectrum of smaller than micro (sub-micron), but not quite nano (smaller than 100 nanometers).

Nanotechnology isn't actually new to cosmetics, nor is the controversy surrounding the use of certain ingredients. For hundreds of years, both men and women used a powder made of hydroxide, carbonate and lead oxide to make their skin appear pale—even white. The end result was lead poisoning. That changed in the 19th century with the introduction of a facial powder made of zinc oxide—the same ingredient used for the past several decades in sunscreens (think of the stereotypical white nose of beach lifeguards). So, any debate pertaining to the use of nanoparticles in cosmetics should be par for the course. In fact, there are now growing concerns about the increased use of active naturals (completely natural organic and botanical-based ingredients) in cosmetics and *their* potential toxicity.

As for nanoparticles—the use of carbon black, as a make-up, actually dates back to the Egyptians; their eyeliner was pretty distinctive, wasn't it? Known as lamp black, women in China and India also used it as an eyeliner and mascara. In July 2004, the FDA approved the use of carbon black (called D&C Black No 2), as a color additive in cosmetics.

From a modern perspective, the first known product to leverage engineered nanotechnology (from Shiseido) apparently became commercially available in 1991, although I haven't been able to track down the specifics. I do know that a decade later, in 2001, Shiseido launched its Elixir foundation, which contained nanoparticles of titanium dioxide and zinc oxide. From my research, it appears that L'Oreal launched (and openly advertised) the first nano-based product in 1997.

Most personal care products leveraging nanotechnology are actually more widely available (and actively marketed) in Europe and Asia. This isn't coincidental; they're by far the largest markets. The US comes in third. Japanese consumers spend the most for personal care products—1.5 times more per capita than US consumers. Plus, it appears that Asian consumers (and their European counterparts), are more open to using new technology.

Case in point, Avon is the leading direct-seller of cosmetics. The company has a few patents pertaining to nanoscale materials, and in late 2005 introduced the Cleawhite C line, which was described as being "nano-formulated." But it's only available in Asia.

It is widely reported that L'Oreal holds one of the most extensive patent portfolios relating to nanotechnology. I also remember something along the lines that about 2,000 patents pertaining to nanotechnology and its use in cosmetics were registered annually (or within a single year, I don't recall which) in Japan. Either way, the bottom line is clear—the cosmetics business is an extremely competitive one, and companies must continually innovate. By design, many products stick around for only a few years; an irritation many women can attest to since they're frequently forced to find replacements for beloved products.

As a marketing-intensive business, the more scientific sounding the product, the better. But as you've learned, there is indeed real science behind those big words. Terminology seems to take two tracks: next-generation ingredients and next-generation ingredient size/delivery mechanisms.

From an ingredient standpoint, buzzwords which probably sound familiar include: Retinol (Vitamin A), Alpha-hydroxy Acids, green tea, Alpha-lipoic Acids, Coenzyme Q-10, copper peptides, soy isoflavones, antioxidants (Vitamin C and Vitamin E), and natural actives (including botanical and organic ingredients). Natural actives range from spice extracts, gums and fruit acids, to vegetable oils, plant extracts and vitamins. They all have specific properties that help to lift, nourish, tighten, etc.

In terms of how these ingredients work their magic, some of the current descriptions of next-generation particle size/delivery methods include: cerasomes, ceraspheres, liposomes, micro-emulsion, micronized, microsomes, microsphere, nano-delivery, nano-encapsulation, nano-vitamin, nanocapsules, nanodispersion, nanoemulsion, nanoencapsulated, nanoliposome, nanoparticles, nanosomes, nanosphere, nanovectors, niosomes, novasomes, oleosomes, ultraspheres and vectorised.

Plus, now there are all sorts of things relating to photonics; words to look for include brightening, interference pigments, photosomes and whitening.

Mind-boggling, isn't it? As you're about to see, trying to sound scientific (in an extremely competitive environment), can open the door to misconception. So, what exactly do these words mean, and why is nano-anything such a big deal?

Let's start with why nanotechnology is such a big deal. The whole point behind cosmetics is the targeted delivery of vitamins, botanicals and other active ingredients into the skin. The smaller their size, the better they're able to penetrate the skin's outer layer in order to moisturize, soften wrinkles, etc.

The skin in made up of three layers: the epidermis, the dermis and the subcutis. The subcutis is the deepest layer and consists of collagen and fat. The thickest layer is the middle, the dermis. Here's where all of the blood vessels, hair follicles, sweat glands, nerves and other structures are found. The epidermis is the outer-most layer. While it's quite thin compared to the other two, it consists of three layers in and of itself. The outermost layer is continuously shed; the middle layer contains living cells that replace the dead ones. The deepest layer, the basal layer, is where new cells are formed.

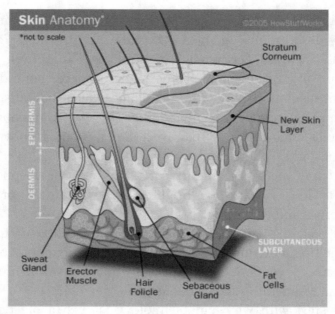

Structure of the skin. Image courtesy of HowStuffWorks.com.

The epidermis is very good at what it's supposed to do—protecting the deeper layers. So, putting lotion on a layer of dead skin cells doesn't seem very effective, does it? But if you could penetrate deeper, then ingredients could be more effective.

Most products are designed to hold moisture in the skin by creating a 'barrier' from external elements. Nanoscale ingredients can penetrate the upper layers of the skin, which improves the appearance of skin by making it plumper and thus more youthful looking. Nanotechnology also makes it possible to use some ingredients (by encapsulating them) that would otherwise cause irritation on their own.

Let's use Vitamin E as an example. It's a sought-after ingredient due to its ability to counteract free radicals (it's an antioxidant), protect against UV damage and reduce inflammation. The biggest issue is that since Vitamin E is hydrophobic (meaning it's repelled by water), adding it to a water-based product really isn't possible. This means that it can only be used in oil-based products, making it difficult to apply or simply not appealing to use. It's going to sit on the skin for a while and feel greasy until it's absorbed.

However, at the nanoscale, Vitamin E disperses evenly into gel, a much more acceptable formulation because it penetrates into the skin a lot faster, leaving the skin feeling soft. As a result, many new cosmetics, and creams and lotions in particular, leverage nanoemulsions to use certain ingredients more effectively.

Sunscreens are another good example. At the microscale, sunscreen agents—titanium dioxide and zinc oxide in particular—are an opaque white; but at the nanoscale, both are nearly translucent. If you think about it, the number of foundations and tinted moisturizers with SPF protection exploded over the past decade; at the same time, these products became lighter feeling and more translucent. That could only be possible with nanoscale materials.

The Science

Going back to our list of unfathomable cosmetic terminology, let's take a quick look at each of these words and what they really mean to the cosmetics you use.

Liposomes

A liposome is basically a vesicle, a sphere that's used to store and transport materials within the body at the cellular level. Think of it as a tiny water balloon, except with the consistency of a soap bubble. In cosmetics, liposomes are widely used to encapsulate ingredients like vitamins to both protect them, and help them better penetrate the skin. They're generally made of lipids (or phospholipids), both of which are fats, which is what our bodies use to store energy. The round objects in the photo at the beginning of this chapter are vesicles.

In most instances (at least according to company patents that I took a look at), liposomes range in size from a few nanometers to a few microns. Most fall within the sub-micron range, which, as pointed out earlier, is not technically nanotechnology, but can certainly be described as nanoscale.

L'Oreal is perhaps best known for their use of liposomes, but other firms who promote the use of liposomes in some products include Christian Dior and Erno Lazlo. As you look through the various terms described in this chapter, it's fairly apparent that many cosmetic terms end with "-somes". As such, it's likely those ingredients are liposomes of some type; the name is simply uniquely branded for that particular company.

Now that you know what a liposome is, let's take a look at the different ways that companies are creating and branding their own version of liposomes:

- Cerasomes/Ceraspheres®—Cerasomes and Ceraspheres® are a type of liposome. Ceramsomes are a ceramic or silica-coated liposome. Developed by Lipoid, Ceraspheres® are a nanoemulsion based on cerasomes.

- Cubosomes—Procter & Gamble is the world's largest manufacturer of personal care products. Some of their brands include Camay, Clairol Herbal Essences, Clairol Nice 'n Easy, Cover Girl, Gillette, Head & Shoulders, Hugo Boss, Ivory, Max Factor, Noxzema, Olay, Old Spice, Pantene, Pert, Safeguard, Secret, Vidal Sassoon, and Zest. The company refers to nanoparticles they've developed as CuboSomes. Although there are few details available, given the name, it's likely that they're a type of liposome.

- I-Spheres™—Developed by Tri-K Industries, I-Spheres™ are essentially the encapsulation of an ingredient to allow for targeted, controlled release. One of their most recent products is Cehami PF, which is extracted from a member of the daisy flower; it has anti-inflammatory and regenerative properties.

- Nanoliposome—A nanoliposome is simply a small liposome, but it's not necessary smaller than 100 nm.

- Nanosome—A nanosome is simply a small liposome, and is a term coined by L'Oreal nearly a decade ago. Although the word isn't trademarked or registered, it appears to be exclusively used by them. L'Oreal is a global cosmetics powerhouse. Some of their brands include Biotherm, Cacharel, Giorgio Armani, Helena Rubenstein, Kérastase, Laboratoires Garnier, Lancôme, Lanvin, L'Oreal, Matrix, Maybelline, Ralph Lauren, Redken, and The Body Shop.

  In 1997, L'Oreal launched Plénitude Futur·e, openly advertising the use of Nanosome technology to deliver Vitamin E to the skin. In 1998, L'Oreal launched RevitaLift Double Lifting (also leveraging Nanosomes). Sometime in mid 2006, L'Oreal removed all mention of nanotechnology from its main international website (most notably its research pages), but regional sites still discuss their use of nanotech approaches, primarily Nanosomes.

- Niosomes™—Lancôme's Niosomes™, which is their version of a liposome, range in size from 100-300 nanometers and deliver ingredients such as Kojic acid and caffeine.

- Novasome—Created by IGI, Novasomes are vesicles generally 200-700 nanometers in size. In keeping with the trend by those within the cosmetic industry to call nanoscale particles a micro-something, the company refers to its technology as microencapsulation.

  Estée Lauder (whose brands include brands include Aramis, Aveda, Bobbi Brown, Bumble and Bumble, Clinique, Darphin, Donna Karan, Estée Lauder, La Mer,

M.A.C., Origins, Prescriptives, Stila, and Tommy Hilfiger), and who has numerous patents referring to nanoscale materials, uses IGI's Novasomes in its Estée Lauder Renutriv and Resiliance lines.

Some products within Johnson & Johnson's Neutrogena brand also use the Novasome technology, although they're difficult to identify.

- Oleosomes—Coined by L'Oreal, Oleosomes range in size from 150-500 nanometers. They're essentially liposomes, except the center is comprised of an oil or oil-based ingredient, rather than a water-based ingredient.

- Ultraspheres®—Developed by Lipoid, Ultraspheres® are a nanoemulsion leveraging liposomes.

- Vectors/Vectorised—In the cosmetic world, vectors are a means of protecting (or basically encapsulating) active ingredients with lipid coatings, and thus improving their delivery into the skin. In other words, they're liposomes. On marketing materials and ingredient lists, look for things like "Vectorised Vitamin E". Lancôme uses this terminology extensively; their vectors include Nano-capsules®, nanoemulsions, and oleosomes. A nano-vector is simply a nanoscale vector.

  Lancôme remains very open about its use of Niosomes™ (first introduced in 1986), Nanocapsules® (launched in 1995 via Primordiale Intense Crème and then in 2002 via Impactive), Nanoemulsions (found in Re-Source in 1996), Nutrispheres™ (for Hydra Zen in 2000), and Oleosomes. All of these approaches fall under the scope of what they call vectors, or vectorised ingredients.

Micronized (aka micro-anything)

Other terms that fit into the cosmetic "micro" modus operandi include: microemulsion, microfine, microsome and microsphere. While conducting a patent search, it became readily apparent that micronized refers to particles ranging in size from a few nanometers to 100 microns. This basically encompasses anything that's micro, sub-micron and nanoscale in size.

Given concerns about the use of nanoscale anything, embracing the word "micronized" could be a smart move on the part of cosmetic firms, but incredibly frustrating when trying to figure out exactly what kind of material is in use—much less its size. While the term proliferated in 2006, a few companies actually *stopped* using it as well, indicating that the reference was a not-so-subtle cover for a nanoscale material.

In general, what I've found is this: the word "fine" generally applies to particles that are microns in size; "microfine" seems to apply to particles that are sub-micron in size; and "ultra-fine" seems to apply to particles that are indeed nanoscale. But, there are always exceptions, and I've found plenty.

In 1999, Procter & Gamble introduced the Oil of Olay Complete UV Protective Moisture Lotion line, which used "microfine zinc oxide" for protection against UVA and UVB rays. The ingredient (called Z-Cote) comes from BASF and is well known to have a particle size smaller than 100 nanometers.

Shiseido, the leading cosmetic firm in Asia, is actively involved in the research and application of nanoscale materials to cosmetics and has even won awards for those efforts. Shiseido is quite open about their nanotechnology research, and announced in late 2004 that they're working with BASF on "micronized zinc oxide" cosmetic formulations for use in sun protection.

Nanodispersion

A nanodispersion is essentially the even distribution of nano-scale ingredients in a liquid, gel or powder.

Nanoemulsion

An emulsion is comprised of two ingredients that don't mix well—like oil and water. Nanoemusions are typically comprised of particles around 50 nanometers in diameter. The use of nano-particles means that the emulsifiers used to bind oil and water are less oily. They not only improve product texture (ie. making it lighter and less sticky), but also allow for product transparency.

Nanoencapsulated

Encapsulation basically means creating an outer layer on another material—a good illustrative example is chocolate candies coated with a hard shell: chocolate on the inside, thin coating on the outside. With nano-encapsulation, that outer layer is just a few nanometers thick. In the case of cosmetics, a microparticle encap-sulated with a nanolayer of some other material is frequently described as both a microparticle and nano-encapsulated, both of which are technically correct.

- Nanocapsules®—At one time Lancôme used the terminology "vitamin nanocapsules" in conjunction with its Soleil line of after sun treatments; they've since replaced that with "vectorised" (see "Vectors" above under "Liposome"). Be careful not to add an "s" when talking about more than one nanocapsule, since the plural form is a registered trade-mark of Lancôme. Nanocapsules® range in size from 100-600 nanometers and deliver the active ingredients Vitamin A and Vitamin E.

Nanoparticle

This was fully discussed in Chapter 3, but it's generally a particle with a diameter of less than 100 nm. In the cosmetics industry, a particle with dimensions of less than 900 nanometers (or 0.9 micrometers) is referred to as both a nanoparticle and a microparticle; in this book I refer to anything smaller than 900 nanometers as being "nanoscale".

- Nanosphere—A nanosphere is a round particle with nanoscale proportions.

Photonics/Photosomes

This category includes words such as brightening, interference pigments, lifting and whitening, all of which is technical speak for playing with the light spectrum of ingredients. In this respect, products provide an optical illusion of skin looking brighter and more youthful. The end result is creating particles that diffuse light in all directions, meaning fine lines are made less visible due to what's basically an optical illusion. Think of the "soft focus" effect that's often used in interviews on TV—you know, that fuzzy look used, particularly when it comes to aging female celebrities (I won't name names but I'm sure you can think of examples).

In addition to being nearly transparent, nanoscale titanium dioxide and zinc oxide also have a whitening effect. This may explain the surge in "brightening", "lightening" and "whitening" products in the past couple of years. It's not about teeth whitening or lightening age spots, but rather, leveraging photonic effects to improve the appearance of skin. Along these lines, in early 2005, Shiseido received top honors at the International Federation of Societies of Cosmetic Chemists for their "reflector powder," a compound of ultra-fine pearlescent pigments and nanocrystals.

Others working on similar photonic techniques include Shu Uemera and Estée Lauder, although particle size is believed to be micro-scale. Even so, it's likely they'll be marketed as "optical rejuvenating powder" (as in the case of Shiseido) or something along those lines. It certainly appears that both nano and sub-micron particles will come into play in these kinds of products.

Anti-Aging/Skincare

Anti-aging products alone accounted for some $50 million in 2005; it is also the fastest growing product segment. Baby boomers, loath to grow old, much less look old, will pay almost anything to remain youthful looking.

Beauty products come and go. Some of those previously available which promoted the use of nanoscience include: Biotherm Age Fitness Nuit, Lancôme Rénergie Morpholift eye cream, Lancôme Soleil Instant Cooling Spritz (nanocapsules), and Vichy Reti C. If you didn't notice already, it's interesting to point out that all of these products fall under the L'Oreal umbrella.

Since more companies are now avoiding the term "nano," even with the alternatives discussed earlier, it's hard to determine where and how it's being used today. So, let's take a look at a short-list of companies and products that openly leverage nano-scale materials (or say that they do), to counteract the effects of aging and/or provide improved skin care.

Amorepacific is the leading cosmetic firm in South Korea. Their Amorepacific line became available in the U.S. in early 2006 at both Bergdorf Goodman and Neiman Marcus. Three of their products are marketed as utilizing the company's Nano-Delivery Technology®, which is described as a *microscopic* encapsulated capture/delivery system: the Time Response Skin Renewal Cream, Time Response Eye Renewal Cream, and Time Response Intensive Skin Renewal Ampoules.

In 2004, Amorepacific entered two products for consideration in the CEW (Cosmetic Executive Women) Beauty Awards. Those were the Skin Energy Hydration Delivery System (a spray-on moisture booster) and the Stabilizing Serum Skin Normalizer; both used the company's Nano-Delivery Technology®.

Chanel sells two body lotions described as nanoemulsions: Chanel No. 5 Sheer Moisture Mist and Coco Mademoiselle lotion.

L'Oreal introduced RevitaLift Double Lifting, one of the first products to make use of the company's Nanosome technology, in 1998; it is still available today, although it's formulated as an Intense Re-Tightening Gel + Anti-Wrinkle Treatment. A refreshed marketing angle is understandable given the fact that it's been on the market for nearly ten years; that's unheard of for cosmetics.

Another product within this line that also makes use of Nano-somes includes the RevitaLift Intense Lift Treatment Mask. Although the RevitaLift cream doesn't specifically state the use of Nanosomes, it was advertised as such in 2002; it's likely that the formulation hasn't changed, just the marketing materials.

La Prairie, a high end skincare regime out of Switzerland, touts the use of a nanoemulsion of Vitamin C in Swiss Alpine water in its Skin Caviar Intensive Ampoule Treatment. The product was entered for consideration in the 2005 CEW Beauty Awards.

Lancôme offers up the most varied mix of technical terms— most of which point to nanotechnology. However, as a subsidiary of L'Oreal, that should come as no surprise. One of their newest products, Platinéum relies on hydroxyapatite, which is basically calcium. Although the packaging describes them as "microscopic molecules" it's intriguing to note that nanoparticles of hydroxy-apatite are now used in next-generation toothpastes (which I discuss later in this chapter).

Here's a list of some the products in which Lancôme currently refers to the use of their nanoscale ingredients in some way:

- BIENFAIT MULTI-VITAL—A moisturizer for the face, one of its listed ingredients is vectorised Vitamin E.

- Body Délisse—A body lotion, it uses Nanocapsules® to deliver ceramides (basically a lipid—fat—that helps retain water) into the skin.

- Caresse—A body lotion, it relies on vectorised Tri-Ceramides to limit dehydration.

- Flash Bronzer Tinted Self-Tanning Moisturizer—This self-tanner contains Nanocapsules® of Vitamin E. In 2005, Lancôme entered its Hydra Flash Bronzer Daily Face Moisturizer in the CEW Beauty Awards for consideration of patented technology or R&D breakthrough. The product leveraged Lancôme's nanocapsule technology.

- Hydra Zen Cream—A moisturizing cream for the face, it contains nano-encapsulated Triceramides (formerly called Nutrispheres™).

- Rénergie Microlift, Rénergie Microlift Neck, Rénergie Microlift Eye, and Rénergie Flash Lifting Serum—All of the products in this line of facial moisturizers rely on Microlifts/Microlifters, which are further described as nano-particles of silica and proteins.

- Sôleil Cool Confort After Sun Rehydrating Face Cream—This product contains vectorised Vitamin E and C.

- Sôleil Cool Confort After Sun Rehydrating Body Milk—This product contains vectorised Vitamin E and C.

- Sôleil Soft-Touch Moisturizing Sun Lotion SPF 15—This product contains vectorised vitamin E.

Color/Make-Up

In 2005, color cosmetics generated a little more than $40 billion in sales worldwide. This particular beauty segment is a key end user of metal nanoparticles; primarily iron oxides (as a pigment) in addition to titanium and zinc (to block UV).

With anti-aging products such as moisturizes, it makes sense to use nanotechnology to deliver ingredients deeper into the skin to hydrate and improve skin texture, as well as make sunblock transparent. But what role does it play with make-up? Nanoscale ingredients help lipstick to last longer, smear less, reflect light and glow in vibrant colors. With foundations and powders, they have a smoother finish, and are much lighter and more translucent.

As an indication of how much more widely accepted nanotechnology is in Asian cosmetics, two firms (aside from Shiseido) launched new products in 2006. The Excellent Day Emulsion Foundation from Noevir is a nano-emulsion, while Kose simply touts the use of "Nanotechnology" in its Rutina nano-force moisturizer and its Rutina nano-white foundation. Speaking of whitening, at one point Christian Dior sold the DiorSnow Pure UV Ultra-Whitening UV Base SPF 30 with "Nano UV filters".

Let's take a look at some of the color cosmetics that are known to make use of nanoscale ingredients.

In mid 2005, when L'Oreal first publicized the development of their new High Intensity Pigments line, the company was open about using "nanoscience to control the color effect". That is, using engineered nanoparticles to produce more vivid colors, as well as iridescent and/or metallic effects. When launched in early 2006, the company simply marketed it as a new photonics technology.

In late 2006, M.A.C. introduced Plushglass lip gloss and volumizer, which uses Nanosomes to deliver phospholipids, as well as soybean and licorice extracts. The bottom line is lip gloss with a super moisturizing formula.

Sally Hansen's Diamond Strength No Chip Nail Color relies on "advanced nanotechnology" and was a 2006 CEW Beauty Awards Insider's Choice Finalist. Another product, Thicken Up!, lists micronized Polycarbonated Resin as an ingredient.

In 2001, Shiseido launched its Elixir foundation, which uses a combination of 10 nm particles of silicon dioxide and zinc dioxide to smooth (and even prevent), dry, rough skin. Shiseido's Pureness Matifying Compact and Benefiance Extra Smoothing Compact are said to use the same technology, although the company simply refers to an exclusive powder ingredient.

The first product to use its award-winning "Reflector Powder" (which minimizes the appearance of shadows that make fine lines more visible), is the Revital Lifting Compact. The technology is used in other products as well.

I want to take a moment to discuss the use of "micronized" ingredients. I believe that there's a high probablility that many of such products are indeed nanoscale; not necessary below 100 nanometers, but certainly within the sub-micron range. One reason for this conclusion is the fact that "micronized" ingredients appear in so few products. I should note that micronized talc is a fairly common ingredient—but it is NOT nanoscale—the particle dimensions are typically a few micrometers in diameter. The use of the term "micronized" in conjunction with minerals, pigments, vitamins and UV agents is what's likely to be nanoscale. Let's take a look at a few examples.

Not too long ago, Biotherm offered Source Therapie Superactiv, a lightweight lotion that was "enriched with micronized pearlizers". As we learned in Chapter 3, Engelhard is a leading supplier of special effect pigments, such as pearlescence, for use in cosmetics.

Pevonia Botanica® is a skin care line generally only sold in spas. Their Ligne Sevactive (Dry Line) utilizes microemulsified Vitamins A, E and C. As we now know, nanotechnology is how

Vitamin E can be added to moisturizers (as evidenced from the profuse use of nanoscale Vitamin E by Lancôme). Several products within Pevonia's line of professional spa body treatments incorporate micronized minerals, algae and seaweed. Two products utilizing micronized titanium dioxide are no longer available.

Laura Mercier sells a Secret Brightening Powder which contains micronized pigments; something very similar to Shiseido's reflector powder, which as noted above, contains ultra-fine pearlescent pigments and nanocrystals.

In late 2000, Revlon launched the Skinlights Color Collection, whose products are formulated with micronized translucent minerals. The Glosslights lip gloss refers to the use of light capturing micro-crystals. The fact that the minerals are translucent certainly seems to suggest the use of nanoscale pigments, since that's a property unique to them.

Deodorant

Both MEMS and nanotechnology are playing a role in deodorants. First, there is one deodorant that I know of that uses a nano-emulsion: NIVEA deodorant PURE Roll-on. While this is the only deodorant example that specifically states its use of nano, I can't help but wonder whether nanomaterials are playing a more extensive role, especially in light of recent formulations that are transparent and leave no white residue. These are the same properties of nanoscale sunscreen agents, so why couldn't the active ingredients in deodorant do the same thing?

In early 2006, Lion Corporation introduced a Ban Powder Spray Deodorant which incorporated their new nanotech drying powder. They simply described it as a way to control moisture levels on sensitive skin. One year later, in early 2007, Lion Corporation re-launched their Ban antiperspirant deodorants as "new Ban". One product in the line, new Ban Deodorant Powder

Spray, leverages their nanotech drying powder, which the company touts as a superior way to absorb moisture.

As for MEMS and deodorant, the first known company to offer a product using the TruSpray™ technology (which I discussed in Chapter 2) is the Sara Lee brand Sanex. Two deoderants, Excel Fresh and Excel Soin, leverage the unique oval packaging. Because of the soft diffusion and the nearly gasless approach, a smaller amount of a more concentrated formula is possible. And it lasts as long as the amount found in a larger, conventional can.

Hair Care

Many patents from the leading personal care firms pertaining to nanoscale materials are actually related to hair. Why? From cleaning, conditioning, styling and coloring, hair takes a beating. And of course, prevention of hair loss is a big deal.

Hair is basically a protein called keratin, the same material as the skin's epidermis and even our fingernails. Each strand of hair typically has three layers: the medulla, cortex and cuticle. The medulla only exists in really large, thick hairs. The cortex is what gives hair its strength and color. If there's no pigment, then you have gray hair. The outermost layer is called the cuticle, which serves to protect the inner layers. If you look at the cuticle under a microscope, it would look a little bit like roof shingles covering the entire strand.

Most hair conditioning products focus on being able to "plump up" the cuticle, much like facial moisturizers aim to "plump up" the epidermis.

Simply being able to study hair at the nanoscale allows companies to develop new products that work better, without necessarily relying on nanoscale materials. For example, products such as conditioners can be developed to work in a specific way (such as uniformly coating each strand of hair), and scientists now have the tools to confirm that such a product indeed works as the company intended.

The biggest benefit of using nanoparticles in hair products is that they're able to penetrate the hair shaft, rather than simply coat it. This is especially important for deep conditioning, or putting moisture back into hair that's become dry from over processing (ie. coloring) and blow dryers, as well as curling and flat irons. Interestingly enough, the ability to penetrate the outer layer of the hair shaft doesn't seem to cause as much concern as penetrating the outer layers of the skin.

Dow Corning offers a number of ingredients for use by hair care firms. They're comprised of a nano-particle size silicone emulsion (Dow calls it a microemulsion) for use in leave-in conditioners, mousse and other hair products. Products include Sunflower Nutrition Water (a spray conditioner), Hair Softening Mousse (a leave-in conditioner in mousse form), and Smoothing Hair Refresher (a spray-on hair softener).

One of the most well-known hair care products to leverage nano-emulsions is the Kérastase Aqua-Oleum® hair treatment, which is only available via professional hair salons and spas. As a L'Oreal brand, products within the Kérastase line are believed to be leveraging their nanotech-based technologies. Oleo Fusion, another professional salon product, relies on nano-emulsions as well. An at-home product, Lipo Recharge, uses liposomes.

One company whose entire line of hair care products leverages nano-emulsions is PureOlogy. From their Hydrate, Volume, Essentials, and NanoWorks Systems, to an extensive range of styling products—such as NanoGlaze™ and NanoWax™—all are touted by the company to leverage advanced nanotechnology.

The NanoWorks® shampoo won a 2007 CEW Beauty Awards Insider's Choice Award. In 2005, PureOlogy's HydrateShampoo® won Allure Magazine's Best of Beauty Editor's Choice award for color-treated hair. Given the company's innovation, it shouldn't come as a surprise that L'Oreal acquired PureOlogy in May 2007; specific details of the deal weren't disclosed.

Other – Your Pets

Since we're talking about hair care, the discussion wouldn't be complete without taking a look at what's available for your pets, right? Rocco and all of his furry friends needn't feel left out, because nanotechnology can give them shiny coats too. A company by the name of avVaa World Health Care Products sells a line of products called derma*lustre*® for horses and pets. The skin and coat treatments utilize nano-fine minerals to deep condition, relieve itchy skin and provide healthy shine.

Sunscreen

Most of the controversy (and concern) regarding nanoparticles in cosmetics is centered on the use of nanoscale zinc oxide and titanium dioxide. The FDA approved the use of both ingredients many, many years ago. One reason for the explosion in their use in recent years is the fact that, at the microscale, these products are white when applied (think of the stereotypically white nose of lifeguards at the beach). At the nanoscale, they're nearly transparent. Also, because titanium dioxide and zinc oxide don't irritate sensitive skin, they're ideals for use in products for babies and kids.

The controversy is how deeply nanoparticles can penetrate into the skin, and if they do, whether or not they're harmful. Let's face it, you can find a study that will support whatever conclusion you want. The bottom line is that it comes down to a "which is worse" scenario—the risks of the nanoparticles themselves or the risks of sun damage and skin cancer?

The leading suppliers of nanoscale UV protection are BASF (who uses Z-Cote from NanoPhase), Advanced Nanotechnology (their product is called ZinClear), Micronisers (whose product is called NanoSun), and Ciba. Ciba's product, Tinosorb M, is referred to as a microparticle; it has a dimension of 200 nanometers.

Few sunblock products actually tout the use of nanoscale ingredients. But given my discussion so far, it's fairly obvious that their use is quite widespread. Only one company openly advertises the use of nanotechnology. Crown Laboratories states the use of nanotechnology (both titanium dioxide and zinc oxide) in its Blue Lizard Baby and Blue Lizard Sensitive sunscreens.

Colorescience uses micronized titanium dioxide and zinc oxide in its Sunforgettable sunscreen. As we've seen throughout this chapter, there's a high probability that it is indeed nanoscale. This product was a 2005 Beauty Awards Finalist due to its unique structure: it's actually a powder that's applied with a brush.

Toothpaste

Brushing, flossing, sensitivity—these are all terms that most people associate with their teeth. From time to time, more than one-third of the population experiences sensitive teeth; that is, exposure to hot or cold food causes pain. This happens when the gum recedes and exposes the root, allowing for what's called the cementum to become eroded. When that happens, the dentin is unprotected and nerves in the pulp signal pain.

Nanotechnology to the rescue! Several toothpastes are now available that decrease teeth sensitivity by utilizing nanoparticles of hydroxyapatite—a calcium mineral found in the dentin—which forms a protective barrier on the teeth.

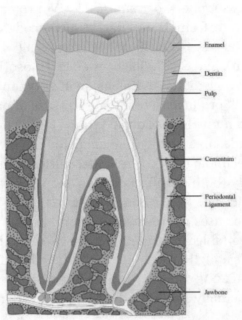

Structure of the tooth. Image courtesy of National Institute of Dental and Craniofacial Research, National Institutes of Health.

Henkel products are probably best known in Europe, but brands familiar to those in the U.S. include Dep, L.A. Looks and Dial soap. Henkel's toothpaste, Nanit®active, consists of nano-crystals of hydroxyapatite and proteins. How it works is that these materials, in conjunction with the saliva in the mouth, encourage the formation of a thin protective layer on the teeth. In essence, the tooth "remineralizes" itself. As a result, tooth sensitivity is reduced (or possibly even eliminated). Nanit®active is available as a gel, paste and tooth strip.

Introduced in 1993 at the low, low price of $24 *per tube*, Sangi's Apaguard M toothpaste "remineralizes" teeth using nanocrystals of hydroxyapatite. (The same approach as Henkel above, but clearly developed nearly a decade earlier). According to Sangi, the toothpaste fills tiny holes on the tooth's surface, essentially repairing teeth and making them stronger. The company licensed its core technology from NASA (the U.S. National Aeronautics and Space Administration).

Launched in April 2002, Clean Clear Plus toothpaste from Kao uses two kinds of fluoride to promote the "recalcification" of teeth and prevent the formation of cavities. Much like Henkel's approach, the result is the formation of a protective layer on teeth. When mixed together in the mouth, the ingredients create particles of calcium fluoride that range in size from 0.005 microns to 1 micron (5 to 1000 nanometers).

Personal Electrics

The category of personal electrics generally includes things like hair dryers and shavers. Most women know that the heat from hair dryers can be damaging to their hair (which is why deep conditioning treatments are so popular). MEMS thermopiles monitor the hair's temperature while drying and help to automatically regulate the heat output.

The new Elevate™ line from Andis (a leading supplier of hair dryers, curling irons and flat irons) features nano-ceramic. They tout it as an ultra-smooth technology that reduces friction—this means the surface of the irons is less likely to catch and break hair.

Why nanoceramic? Metal curling irons can be incredibly damaging; anyone who's used them knows what burning hair smells like. With the move to flat irons in the 1990s, word spread like wildfire that the more costly ceramic versions were much better. Not only because they got hot faster, but they were far less likely to damage your hair. As a result, the switch from metal to ceramic in hair dryers and flat irons is a big deal for all involved.

Nanoceramic coatings are already in use to reduce friction and prevent corrosion in heavy duty applications like military equipment and car engines. While friction reduction in a flat iron probably isn't terribly critical, it is helpful, since their sole purpose is to flatten the cuticle to create super shiny hair. Reducing friction lessens the chance of hair damage.

One of the most interesting uses of nanomaterials is in shavers. In 2004, Philips introduced the Norelco Cool Skin shaver, which uses the Nanoflex™ stainless steel strip from Sandvik in several key shaver components: the stationary cutter head, the rotating cutter knife and the hair lifter.

Philips and Sandvik worked together for about three years to develop the unique nanostructured metal. Key criteria included the ability to be used in conjunction with shaving cream and then cleaned in running water, in addition to being corrosion-resistant, strong and formable (the ability to be fashioned or produced into different shapes).

Philips subsequently launched the Quadra Action and Sensotec shavers using the same steel. It's believed that most shavers on the market today now use this material, such as the Wilkinson Sword FX Diamond Razor and Panasonic's Arc with Vortex Cleaning System WetDry Shaver.

Some of Philips' shavers also have small polymer OLED displays to illustrate the battery's remaining life so you know when it needs to be re-charged.

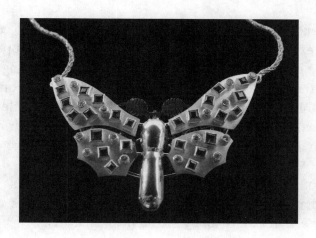

9 • CLOTHING/ACCESSORIES

Like many products that are part of our every-day life, Teflon®
started out as a scientific accident. Since its creation in 1938 by Du
Pont, this non-stick wonder material—technically called polytetra-
fluoroethylene (PTFE)—is probably best known for its use in
cookware via the SilverStone® brand name. But did you know
that Teflon is what gives Gore-Tex® fabrics their unique water
repellency? It's simply a Teflon-treated synthetic fiber.

Despite some reports to the contrary, there's nothing nanoscale
about Teflon. Rather, it's comprised of three layers; each of which
are about 100 microns thick.

A second well-known fabric treatment is 3M's Scotchgard®.
Yet another accidental discovery, it was first marketed in 1956. In
1973, Scotchgard became widely used as a stain-resistant treatment
for carpets. As with Teflon, there's no nano here either.

Neither Teflon nor Scotchgard were purposefully created to provide textiles with anti-stain properties. It just so happened that they were useful for that. Both basically work by coating the fiber to make them hydrophobic—water beads up and rolls off. But the basic problem is that they also made fabrics feel a little stiff. So, they're really good for things like the material on your couch, or jackets and tents, but not ideal for the pants or shirts that you generally wear everyday.

In 1998, the next-generation of fabric treatments made its debut. That's when textile giant Burlington Industries took a 35 percent stake in a start-up by the name of Nano-Tex.

Next-Generation Textile Properties

Nano-Tex has almost single-handedly revolutionized the textile industry. Its various treatments work their magic while allowing fabric to breathe, and more importantly, without changing how the fabric feels; it's still soft, not at all stiff. How exactly it does this is a closely guarded secret, but it's based on the use of what the company refers to as nanowhiskers.

In that respect, the technology works sort of like a peach. Think about that for a moment. A peach has a very light layer of fuzz that you can barely see. But if you sprinkle water on it, it will typically just bead up and roll right off. The company currently offers four treatments: Coolest Comfort, Resists Spills, Repels and Releases Stains and Resists Static.

- Coolest Comfort—With this fiber treatment, moisture is drawn away from the skin and dries quickly, so your body temperature stays better balanced. Depending on the outside temperature, damp clothing can make you hot or cold.

- Resists Spills—The original fiber treatment, liquids typically bead up and simply roll off the fabric or are easily wiped off the surface.

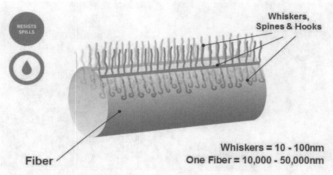

How Resists Spills works. Illustration courtesy of Nano-Tex, Inc.

- Repels and Releases Stains—This fiber treatment generally makes fabrics spill repellant, meaning liquids will roll off; even better, any stains you do get (like a grass or dirt stain on the knees), are easily washed out.

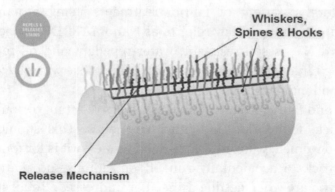

How Repels and Releases Stains works. Illustration courtesy of Nano-Tex, Inc.

- Resists Static—An intriguing fiber treatment, this eliminates static in synthetic fabrics; so when you pull off that stocking hat during dry winter weather, your hair won't stand on end from static electricity.

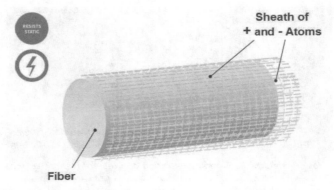

How Resists Static works. Illustration courtesy of Nano-Tex, Inc.

More than 80 textile mills and 100 apparel brands already use these products in countless clothing lines. It's no longer a matter of who's using Nano-Tex treatments; but rather, who's *not*.

But Nano-Tex isn't alone in their innovation. Toray Industries also offers a variety of fabric treatments using a nano-scale processing technique they refer to as NanoMATRIX™. One fabric, Tapguard NT, is soil-resistant, water-repellant and oil-repellant; it's being targeted for use in uniforms, like those worn by workers in the food industry.

A second fabric, Rougeoff, makes fabrics resistant to stains such as lipstick, foundation and other cosmetics. This should really appeal to women, who know first-hand how easy it is for foundation and lipstick to accidentally rub off on clothes—no matter how careful you are when getting dressed or undressed. Retail stores in particular could benefit since their stock won't be ruined as women try clothing on.

A slightly different approach comes from Inkmax. They've developed nano-fine adhesive polymers (about 70 nanometers thick) that are formed on the surface of cotton fabric. Because these polymers attract pigments, they allow for ink jet printing with virtually no water. Using nanoparticle-based ink in conjunction with the nanolayer produces really vivid colors—and it's highly color fast. They're touting it as a unique dying process, rather than an alternative to the screenprinting of graphics on clothing. But both applications actually make sense.

Anti-bacterial is Big

As explained in Chapter 3, the vast majority of silver treatments on the market today are NOT nanotechnology. The X-Static Fiber from Noble Silver Technologies is a silver-coated nylon, which is micro-scale at this point. The use of X-Static is extensive; it's currently licensed to more than 300 companies, including adidas, Danskin, Johnson & Johnson, Malden Mills, Performance Sports Apparel and Puma.

A second approach is the use of zeolites, such as the highly successful product from Agion Technologies, which, as explained earlier, doesn't appropriately fall under the nanotechnology umbrella either. Along those lines, there are several other companies with similar zeolite-based products, including Nisshinbo Industries, who uses copper ions instead of silver ions.

A third approach is the use of actual nanoparticles of silver. NanoHorizons is a leader in this respect with their SmartSilver™ brand, which they offer for integration by textile mills and garment manufacturers. Some of the mills using the technology include Carolina Cotton Works and United Knitting. Another company, CMI Enterprises, is using silver nanoparticles in their own line of soft vinyl upholstery fabrics.

But silver isn't the only nanoparticle being added to fibers; it turns out that nanoparticles of titanium dioxide are useful too. Japan Exlan now offers a fiber called Selfclear, which relies on nanoparticle of titanium oxide to provide deodorizing, antibacterial and soil-resistant properties by catalytic action of light. That is, sunlight causes a self-cleaning effect, much like the window coatings discussed in Chapter 6. A second company, Nishijin Shenshoku uses the same approach; the TioTio air catalyst from Sunward Shokai provides yarn with a deodorizing/antibacterial treatment and relies on the use of titanium oxide to do so.

Completely New Fibers

Beyond coatings and treatments, entirely new fibers are also being developed. One such product is a yarn based on nanoparticles of bamboo charcoal, which has both antimicrobial and deodorizing properties; it's available from Greenyarn.

Japan Wool Textile sells a line called Nikke Miracle products, some of which are nanotech-based. They include:

- Wel Warm—Wool that's treated with nanotechnology to give it moisture-absorbing and heat-generating properties.
- Bambool—A mixture of wool and bamboo fiber that's antibacterial, deodorant and moisture absorbent/releasing.
- CoolTwist—A combination of wool and yarn infused with ceramic nanopowder to block UV rays.

Of all the new fibers I've come across so far, Teijin's MORPHO-TEX® is one of the coolest. As discussed in Chapter 3, it produces an iridescent effect without the use of pigments. The fiber is comprised of 61 layers of polyester and nylon; each is just a few nanometers thick and has a different refractive index. That means each layer is some variation of red, blue, green or yellow. The color you ultimately see also depends of viewing angle and light intensity. According to the company, one of the biggest applications for the fiber is denim.

Impact Resistance

No question one of the most interesting developments pertaining to textiles is what's been referred to as "liquid armor." Called Shear Thickening Fluid (STF), it's a nanoparticle-based coating material which, under normal conditions, allows fabric to remain flexible. However, upon impact, it becomes hard. Developed at the University of Delaware's Center for Composite Materials, in partnership with the Weapons and Materials Research Directorate of the US Army Research Laboratory, they licensed it to Armor Holdings for use in body armor vests, helmets and gloves.

Several other companies have products that work in a similar way, but are based on slightly different technologies.

A company by the name of d3o sells a material made of "intelligent molecules" that is quickly being incorporated into sports gear (see Chapter 10 for numerous examples). It's available as a thin, flexible sheet (designed to conform to the body part it's meant to protect) that vaguely reminds me of bubble wrap. The secret is a viscose fluid and a polymer; under normal conditions, it's flexible, but upon impact, the molecules lock, creating a rigid pad. Given the focus on molecular properties, it sounds like nanoparticles are being put to use.

In early 2007, Dow Corning introduced their Active Protection System. Like STF, it's a coating. In this case, Dow applies silicone to a special, three dimensional "spacer textile support" that's a few millimeters thick. The exact particle size of the silicone is unknown, so I'm not entirely sure if their particular approach is considered nanotech or not. However, given Dow's known work in the area, it's certainly a possibility, especially in light of the above approaches. The first application of the technology is available via

Rukka, who sells a motorcycle riding suit with patches of the material on high-impact areas such as the knees, shins, elbows, shoulders, chest and back.

Propex Fabrics sells a material with excellent impact resistant properties called Curv®, which was developed at the University of Leeds. The end result here is one of a self-reinforcing composite made of polypropylene (PP). That is, the filler material is the same as the matrix material. How they do this is via a process called hot compaction, which controls the molecular orientation of the polymer. Once the fibers are aligned, the surface is melted to hold them in place. This material is stronger and much lighter than conventional PP fabrics. The addition of carbon nanotubes should improve its temperature stability, making it suitable for automotive uses, such as inner door panels and underfloors.

One of the most high-profile applications to date is a new line of luggage from Samsonite, which they introduced in early 2007. The outer shell of their new X'Lite suitcase, which is part of the Black Label line, is made of the Curv® material. This is an ideal use since the most desirable properties of a suitcases is that it's both lightweight and highly impact resistant.

Athletic Apparel

Athletic wear is a natural fit for treatments that wick away moisture (drawing liquid such as sweat away from your skin so it can evaporate) and/or control odor. Only a few companies openly state "nano" something or other in conjunction with their product, but I'm sure there's *a lot* more; just look for moisture wicking and "stay cool" properties.

Here are just a couple of examples that openly mention the use of nanotechnology in some way:

- New Balance created the Skye Crop (a sports bra) for women which makes use of "nano channel yarn" as part of its Lightning Dry™ Extreme liner.
- Yocum activewear, part of the Performance line from adidas, uses the Coolest Comfort technology from Nano-Tex™ to wick away moisture and keep you feeling cool and dry. Pieces in the line include men's and women's shorts, ¾ pants, and capris.

Sportswear

Sportswear is ideal for anti-spill and anti-stain treatments. What I find so interesting in this respect is that the vast majority of garments that currently have these properties are pants and shirts for *men*. Apparently, men are just naturally inclined to spill on themselves; so, the garments below must be a godsend.

- Eddie Bauer—products include Nano-Tex™ Relaxed Fit and Classic Fit shirts, Short and Long Sleeve Performance Polos, Chinos (Classic Fit, Comfort Waist, and Relaxed Fit), and Khakis (Relaxed Fit, Classic Fit, Comfort Waist, and Slim Fit), and Wrinkle-Resistant Oxford shirts, to name just a few.
- Gap—Stressfree khakis
- Lee—LPK Double Pleat and Plain Front Pant
- LL Bean—Double L® Chinos and Timberledge Pants
- Nordstrom—Smartcare Pique Polos

Hartwell Classic Apparel sells two long-sleeve shirts with a spill and stain-resistant property called Nanocote™. In this case, nanoparticles are evenly distributed over textile fibers to provide a protective layer so liquids bead up and roll off (or are wiped away).

Separates/Suits

In the fall of 2005, Hugo Boss revealed the use of the Nano-Tex Resists Spills treatment in its Orange label men's front-button woven shirts; Paul Stuart offered a line of wool trousers with the same treatment for sale in Japan.

Nano-Tex extended its reach into men's suits in late 2006. Perry Ellis and Hart Schaffner Marx integrated the Resist Spills treatment into their fall 2006 line of men's suits and separates. Sold via Macy's, the Perry Ellis suits are available in seven different styles, with the separates available in four styles. Nordstrom carries the "Traveler" line of Hart Schaffner Marx suits, which is available in two styles.

Outerwear

The use of nanotechnology in outerwear—such as jackets and accessories like gloves—has gotten really interesting lately. Turtle Fur, a leading manufacturer of clothing for cold-weather sports, is integrating NanoHorizons' SmartSilver™ in hats and other garments that will be available for sale in 2007. Water repellence for these kinds of clothes also makes sense (as does anti-static), but anti-pollen? Absolutely.

Anti-Pollen

During 2006, three companies (all Japanese no less) introduced fabrics relying on nanotechnology to make them anti-pollen. That is, pollen grains can't stick to them. Toray Industries led this trend by introducing Anti-Pollen NT in 2005. If by chance a pollen grain does manage to stick to the fabric, it's easier to brush off. So, why is this a big deal?

Take a look at the photo below, which is a mix of all sorts of common pollens, including ragweed. With these prickly kinds of structures it's easy to see why pollen sticks so readily to clothes. For people with allergies, this can be a problem. Maybe not so much while you're walking (since you can't avoid breathing in pollen), but at least you know that it can reduce the level of pollen in your home after being outdoors by brushing off your clothes before going inside the house.

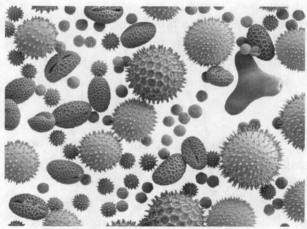

A mix of common pollen grains. Copyright 2007 © RMF/Scientifica/Visuals Unlimited.

Goldwin's Pollen Guard fabric relies on a nanoscale coating. Seven jackets made of the fabric are sold under the Canterbury of New Zealand, Champion, Danskin, Ellesse, Helly Hansen, Laterra and The North Face brand names—but only in Japan, where Goldwin has the rights to sell them. Mizuno Corp. has an anti-pollen fabric for sportswear (such as walking or jogging suits) that it sells via its Superstar brand. Sportswear firm Asics also sells clothing made with an anti-pollen fabric, but these garments are also only available for sale in Japan.

Anti-Static

Land's End is one the first companies to promote the use of the Nano-Tex Resists Static treatment in their ThermaCheck® line of fleece scarves, gloves, and caps. But the property should be fairly easy to recognize in similar items from other companies.

Water Repellence

New Balance Performance Outerwear integrated the Nano-Tex Repels and Releases Stains treatment in a new line of outerwear that became available in the fall of 2006. As a result, the Circa V line of parkas, puffer coats, bomber jackets, down vests and Bog coats, for both men and women, are both liquid-repellant and stain-resistant—features that are important for coats.

Swimwear

In 2006 Toray Industries introduced a brand-new fabric that prevents sand from sticking to swimsuits. It's called, appropriately enough, Sandproof™.

Geologists define sand as rock with a diameter somewhere between 1/16th of one millimeter and 2 millimeters. If you took a handful of sand and looked under a microscope, what you would find is that sand is irregularly shaped. In addition, it's made up of microscopic bits of all sorts of things like coral, sea shells, lava, volcanic rock, quartz and other minerals—depending on the beach you scooped it up from—few of which are perfectly round and smooth. This angular shape is probably why sand sticks to fabric so well. Fortunately, it doesn't have the prickly points like pollen; or else we probably wouldn't be able to walk on it.

Toray's technology does have some water repellent characteristics. Since there's a lot of sand in seawater, it would make sense that the sand would come off with water—sort of like the self-cleaning windows discussed in Chapter 6. But it does also prevent the adhesion of sand itself. It's a great application—how annoying is it to come back home (or to your hotel room) from a day at the beach—and your swimsuit still has sand in it? Not to mention your towel, wet suit and any other textiles you had with you.

Footwear

Greenyarn sells a fairly extensive range of socks based on their bamboo charcoal fiber, which is a great application for this particular technology and a nice alternative to silver. In late 2006, Polar Wrap introduced the ToastyFeet shoe liners, which are made of the highly insulating aerogels; they really do prevent your feet from getting cold in winter weather. It's probably one of the most useful applications of nanotechnology I've come across yet.

In fact, three leading boot manufacturers now incorporate the material (from Aspen Aerogels) right into the boot itself. Two winter/snow boots, the Radiator (from Vasque, part of Red Wing Shoe Company) and the Scrambler (from Salomon), both leverage aerogels in the sole. A line of safety boots created by Heckel Sécurité and UVEX not only has incorporated aerogels into the sole and the boot liner, but there's an aerogel-based insole as well.

Jewelry

If you like diamonds, silver or watches, MEMS and nanotechnology have you covered. Or I should say that you could simply look at your wrist or the jewelry you're wearing to see examples of MEMS and nanotech in action.

Diamonds

Cubic Zirconia, officially called zirconium oxide (ZrO_2), shook up the jewelry industry in the 1980s. Suddenly, "diamonds" were no longer out of reach for anything other than engagement rings and the wealthy. Now "diamond" stud earrings and a tennis bracelet—two hot items at the time—were available for much less than what a real version would cost.

What is so appealing about CZ is that it is virtually undistinguishable from the real thing. Some of the most apparent differences to the trained eye are that CZ is not as hard as a diamond, it's virtually flawless and colorless, and also weighs more than 1.5 times as much.

Today, other means of creating diamonds have leading diamond firms like DeBeers on the defensive, and nanotechnology is smack dab in the middle. As with CZ, these stones are flawless, and have the potential to cost far less than the real thing.

Apollo Diamond creates their diamonds in a way that's very similar to cultured pearls. They start with a tiny diamond chip and then use chemical vapor deposition (CVD)—a technique used in the production of semiconductors—to "grow" a diamond, atom by atom. The result is a diamond that is absolutely pure, and colorless. The difference between this "cultured" diamond and a mined one is extremely difficult to detect.

A second company, Gemesis, takes a different approach. They essentially crush carbon under enormous pressure at incredibly high heat until it crystallizes; this results in what appears to be a very rare, yellow diamond.

While the products of both companies clearly have application as jewelry, and they're definitely pursuing this, their main focus is actually electronics; the possibilities across every major market segment are virtually endless.

Silver

A coating developed by Beneq, called nSilver®, made its debut in early 2007. Just 10 nanometers thick, it protects silver from tarnishing. Even better, it's completely transparent, so it doesn't affect the color of whatever silver object it's protecting. One of the largest jewelry firms in Finland, Kalevala Koru, is already using the nanocoating on the silver jewelry it manufactures.

Watches

If your watch has a barometer function, you're almost certainly wearing a MEMS pressure sensor on your wrist. Another way to use these pressure sensors is for navigation through different functions and screens of more complicated watches, like the Tissot T-Touch. You just touch different places of the bezel in order to obtain information on various features.

In early 2005, Patek Philippe created quite a stir in the watch-making industry when they introduced the first Swiss lever escapement with a silicon escape wheel. Traditional steel escape wheels work in conjunction with ruby pallet jewels, and they need to be lubricated because of the "ratcheting" involved. Silicon was heralded as a watchmaking breakthrough because it not only eliminated the need for lubrication, but offered long-term reliability (no need for re-lubrication as the oil seeped away).

Another plus was the fabrication process of the part itself—it could be done in a single step—via micromachining. The method used was deep reactive ion etching (DRIE). Steel escape wheels require up to 50 production steps. With such a small part, there's a lot of room for error given the precise tolerances required for such a tiny device. The lever was housed in a limited edition "Patek Philippe Advanced Research" 39mm Annual Calendar watch, only 100 of which were made.

The next year, Patek Philippe released a second limited edition "Patek Philippe Advanced Research" which incorporated another technical innovation, the Spiromax® balance spring. The spring is what dictates the number of ticks per second, per hour and per day. Its ability to expand and contract, uniformly, as its being wound and unwound, is critical. Since it's made of steel, it can be affected by magnetic fields and temperature, and even rust.

A silicon spring doesn't need to be adjusted for each individual movement, and won't rust, but more importantly, it's isochronous (i.e. has perfect vibration), regardless of temperature, orientation of the movement or presence of magnetic fields. Plus, it's also three times thinner than conventional balance springs. This could open the door to a whole new generation of super-thin watch movements and other components.

Nanotechnology is also slowly making its way into watches via the use of organic light emitting displays (OLEDs). As with cell phones, they're currently limited to just one or two lines of text, but that should change shortly with the development of larger, full-color displays. Watch for a MEMS-based display for watches in the not-too-distant future.

Other

Have you been wondering about the photograph of the butterfly pendant at the beginning of this chapter and what it has to do with MEMS or nanotechnology? This beautiful piece of jewelry, created by Sensory Design & Technology, doubles as a perfume diffuser. Hidden inside are a wireless humidity sensor and a lab-on-a-chip, which work together to deliver fragrance while wearing it. I thought it was one of the more creative end-uses of MEMS that I've ever come across.

Tattoos

I included a discussion about tattoos in this chapter, because as a personal adornment, I think they're better classified as an accessory, rather than a cosmetic. Nanotechnology and tattoos? From what you've read so far in this book, you shouldn't be too surprised by now; the connection is actually quite ancient.

Tattooing is a global tradition that's taken place for thousands of years. Attitudes vary about tattoos, and the people who get them. There are any number of reasons why someone might get a tattoo, but in modern society today, the impetus seems to be that it's simply a way of providing a personal statement of who you are or what you're about.

The tattooing process itself ranges from hand tapping ink into the skin via sharp sticks, animal bones, bamboo or steel, to an oscillating array of needles. It seems to me that there's potential here for the use of MEMS needles.

As for the tattoo inks, here's where it gets interesting. Pigments used range from titanium dioxide and iron oxides to carbon black and other dyes. As we already know, carbon black is a naturally-occurring nanoparticle, and both titanium dioxide and iron oxides are now being used at the nanoscale in cosmetics.

But wait, there's more. Want a tattoo but aren't so sure about having it forever? Have a tattoo but aren't so keen on the cost (and pain) involved with getting it removed? A start-up by the name of Freedom-2 may have the answer: tattoo ink that allows for tattoos to be both permanent *and* easily removable.

The company starts with biodegradable and bioabsorbable pigments, such as cosmetic-grade iron oxide, and then encapsulates them into a clear, polymer, nanoscale bead. Tattoo artists don't need special equipment to use this ink; the only difference is the structure of the actual ink particles.

Because the ink is encapsulated in polymethymethacrylate (PMMA), the tattoo is removable via a single, standard laser treatment. The laser causes the polymer to break up, allowing the pigment to be resorbed by the body. As a result, tattoos created with this ink are indeed permanent, yet much more easily removed than those created with conventional tattoo ink. The ink became available in early 2007.

Freedom-2 is also developing a bead that allows the pigments to slowly disperse, so that the tattoo will simply disappear over a period of time.

By the way, the FDA hasn't *technically* approved the use of any ink for tattoos; but that's not really a big deal since the pigments used to create the inks (as well as color cosmetics) are.

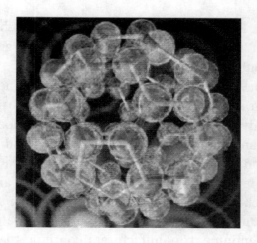

10 • RECREATION/SPORTS

Who knew that something as innocuous as ski wax would forever change sports? The launch of Nanowax (from Nanogate) in 2000 was the proverbial "shot heard 'round the world" and one that heralded the introduction of nanotechnology in sporting goods. The next four years saw the introduction of various materials for various sports, each of which caused ripples due to their increasing levels of ingenuity.

In 2001, Wilson Racquet, a division of Wilson Sporting Goods, introduced a revolutionary new tennis ball, the Wilson Double Core, which used the Air D-Fense technology developed by InMat. This nanoclay composite was used to coat the inner core of tennis balls; the result was that they retained air better than rubber, and thus lasted longer. The following year (2002), saw one of the first uses of Teijin's MORPHOTEX® nanofiber—Descente North America created skiwear with the fiber for the 2002 Swiss Winter

Olympic team. Fullerenes made their commercial debut in 2003 in bowling balls. Two years later, carbon nanotube-enhanced bike frames were put to use in the Tour de France.

Materials have long played an important and somewhat controversial role in sports equipment. Anything that can give you a competitive advantage is fair game, so long as it doesn't give you an unfair advantage. Controversy seems to go hand in hand with the introduction of new materials; at least until they can be evaluated and deemed fair game. Real scientific advances are one thing, stuffing a baseball bat with cork is another matter entirely.

This is really turning out to be an ideal realm for nano-composites. Equipment manufacturers continue to seek ways to make equipment both lighter and stronger, and nanomaterials can do just that. The leader is this respect is Easton Sports; they've literally taken the carbon nanotube-based NanoSolve® material from Zyvex and run with it in key areas such as baseball and cycling. Others are now quickly following suit with nano-composites, but not necessarily those made of carbon nanotubes.

As for MEMS sensors, their use hasn't been terribly extensive to date. MEMS pressure sensors have a long history of use in SCUBA gear, and accelerometers have found their way into the world of sports as well—particularly for use in training systems. But as the age of electronics creeps its way into recreational equipment of all kinds, MEMS are there, front and center—some really innovative approaches are in play.

Astronomy

Stargazing is a great activity for kids and adults alike. Until recently, you either had to rely on your own knowledge of constellations, or use star charts to help you find the planet you're looking for and identify other celestial objects that you can't quite figure out what they are.

In 2006, Celestron introduced the SkyScout™. About the size of a can of soda, you hold it up to the night sky and with the help of GPS it quickly identifies pretty much any celestial object you point it at. Or, it can help you search for specific constellations or planets. While looking through it (much like a camera), an outer ring in the view finder has little red lights that help pinpoint the exact location of say, a planet, by indicating that you need to move the device left, or up. The system can then provide information about what it is you're looking at, via text or audio. Two MEMS accelerometers work as an inclinometer (to gauge tilt) and provide the system with its easy-to-use "point and shoot" interface.

MEMS deformable mirrors are also playing a role in the adaptive optics (AO) systems in big telescopes, like those used in research observatories. They work by correcting for variations in the atmosphere, so these ground-based telescopes can achieve much better image clarity. With the Hubble Telescope rapidly aging, improving the imaging capabilities of other telescopes is becoming even more important to our ability to "see" the universe and all of its wonders.

Badminton/Racquetball/Squash

I don't generally consider badminton to be the kind of sport where stronger, lighter racquets are necessary, since the birdie (technically called the shuttlecock) doesn't weigh nearly as a much as a racquetball (nor is it hit nearly as hard), and the racquets weigh nearly nothing to begin with. But four leading suppliers of badminton equipment have already moved to the use of nano-materials for improved racquet stiffness and power.

HEAD announced the development of its first badminton line in late 2006, which includes HEAD Metallix racquets, which will be available in the summer of 2007. They use nanometal from PowerMetal Technologies to create a "nanocrystalline reinforcement layer" to provide added stiffness to the neck (the longest part) of the racquets.

PROTECH offers several badminton racquets with a "nano power frame technology" that uses Hi Modulus graphite and nano carbon. Products include the Max Nano 9900, Max Nano 8000, Nano Titanium 9000, Max Nano 8800, Max Nano 7800, Max Nano 7000, and Max Nano 6000.

Wilson offers the nCode Badminton Racquet, the nRage racquet-ball racquet, and the n120 squash raquet (which replaces the n145), all of which use their nCode technology. Here, "nano-sized silicon dioxide crystals permeate the voids between the carbon fibers." The result is a racquet that's "2x stronger, 2x more stable, and up to 22 percent more powerful."

Yonex uses both its Elastic Ti technology (a nanoscale titanium alloy) and NANOSCIENCE (a composite comprised of nano-sized particles of fullerene and carbon), to create their next-generation badminton racquets. Racquets include the Nanospeed 9000, Nanospeed 8000, Nanospeed 7000, and Nanospeed 6000.

Baseball/Softball

A baseball (and softball) bat is far more complicated than you might think. It's not just a stick to hit a ball. It's been carefully designed to provide a quick, powerful, balanced swing. The term "sweet spot" applies to the part of the barrel that's considered the best spot to hit the ball. Where exactly that is depends on the bat's construction. Reducing a bat's weight can increase hitting power, which is why wood bats are sometimes found to be corked—or filled with cork. Since metal bats are allowed in amateur baseball, manufacturers are constantly on the lookout for new materials that will improve hitting with a bat that weighs less. Nanomaterials offer these kinds of properties.

In 2005, Easton Sports unveiled a new line of baseball and softball bats using its carbon nanotube (CNT) nanocomposite in the handle. The advantages were "optimized flex and responsiveness." At the same time, the company ran a series of television ads; the first known to actually say "carbon nanotube."

The following year, in 2006, Easton Sports introduced its next-generation line of bats for baseball and softball, this time expanding the use of its nanocomposite. The Stealth Comp CNT bats rely on the nanocomposite from the handle to the barrel, "creating one of the largest sweet spots ever." The line includes baseball bats for adults, youth, as well as both slow-pitch and fast-pitch softball. Another sports manufacturer, Worth, introduced and sold a line of baseball and softball bats (called the Asylum Nano Composite) in 2006, but they're no longer available.

Boating/Yachting

One wouldn't think that technology could play much of a role in boating, but as it turns out, that couldn't be further from the truth. Known applications at this time range from cushions and stabilization systems to compasses and the materials used in the construction of sailing yachts.

Antenna/Boat Stabilization

Thanks to MEMS, a number of boating systems have become increasingly sophisticated; while these were originally developed for use by the military, cost and availability is such that the recreational boats are now benefiting as well. Naval ships were among the first to use MEMS gyros to stabilize communications antennas. Today, leisure boats can apply the same technology to their satellite TV antennas. Ship movement can cause fairly significant rocking of antennas, which disrupt the reception of satellite signals.

MEMS gyros can help to minimize that problem, and thus maintain signal integrity. They do so by compensating for the subtle rotational "wiggle" of antennas caused by water movement.

Taking this application a step further, MEMS gyros are also part of stabilization systems that reduce the rolling motion caused by waves. This is just starting to make its way into large, commercial ships and boats that tend to spend a lot of time at sea, but with the continued reduction of gyro prices, it's starting to be considered for leisure craft as well.

Compass

Yet another military use of MEMS sensors is finding its way into commercial and recreational boats: electronic compasses. Here, MEMS magnetic sensors and accelerometers are combined to provide dead reckoning capabilities, just like with personal GPS systems. In this case, the compass provides precise heading, as well as roll and pitch data for attitude measurement. You could even connect a pressure sensor to the system for water depth data.

Cushions/Seat Vinyl

CMI Enterprises is a leading supplier of the soft vinyl fabric used for boat cushions (amongst many other end-uses). They've recently introduced NBT™ Marine, a coating that leverages nanotechnology so that the fabric is not only spill and stain resistant, but has UV protection. The latter is especially important. Have you ever seen really seen nice, dark seat cushions on a boat? The sun can be harsh; not only making the vinyl too hot to sit on, but also rapidly fading it. This is a common problem no matter where you boat—whether it's Minnesota or the Mediterranean—but how nice is it to now have boat seats and cushions that don't visibly fade in a short period of time?

Sailing Mast

In October 2006, Synergy Yachts introduced the 350RL, whose mast (the tall pole that the sail is attached to) is constructed with carbon fiber and a carbon nanotube composite. Using a nano-composite gives the mast added strength and stiffness, without adding weight. The yacht also uses a nanoparticle-based paint, called Nanoblack™, on the bottom of the outer hull; it provides improved resistance to abrasion and marine growth below the waterline—two things that can affect both speed and performance. At the time of the announcement, Synergy also mentioned the construction of a keel foil with the nanocomposite (it's the big fin attached to the bottom of the boat to help keep it upright), but it is not indicated as such on the specs for the 350RL.

Teak Decks/Furniture

Are you lucky enough to have a boat with wood decks made from teak? Maybe you have teak furniture on your boat. If you do, then you know that the sun and salt water can wreak havoc on this wood. Well, you shouldn't be surprised that a nanotechnology-based solution is now available to help extend the longevity of teak. Teak Guard® Marine is a coating that provides water repel-lence (while maintaining a non-slip finish), and UV protection (so the wood won't turn gray), as well as stain resistance (with food stains being a target here).

Bowling

In 2003, American Bowling Service introduced the Nanodesu X bowling ball, which was one of the first sporting good products to benefit from the use of fullerenes. That particular ball is no longer available, but three others are: Nanodesu Blue, Nanodesu Scarlet and Nanodesu Noble. The use of fullerenes as part of the outer clearcoat provides better protection against chipping and cracking.

But it also has the potential to improve play. The coating makes the ball more slippery in waxed areas of the lane, and curve in non-waxed areas of the lane, so it's possible that players could throw more strikes. I didn't know that the waxing of bowling alley lanes was such an art.

Bullriding

Bullriding? You bet. In 2006, Winnercomm (the largest independent provider of programming for ESPN), created a hockey puck-sized gadget containing a MEMS inertial sensor, which was placed on rodeo bulls to help enhance the viewer experience of ESPN bull-riding coverage. By transmitting the G-forces felt by the rider (via the acceleration and deceleration of the bull), an animated bar chart was able to graphically depict the bull's power.

This isn't the first time ESPN relied on MEMS sensors to enhance the judging of sports events. Back in 2003, ESPN revealed that an accelerometer had been used for timing and scoring in many of the timber events that were part of their Great Outdoor Games (GO Games). It was able to measure the exact moment chopping began and ended; results were then fed directly into scoring computers.

Cycling

Bike manufacturers are continually innovating so they can offer the latest and greatest in materials that will achieve the optimal balance between strength, weight, stiffness, riding comfort, and durability. The first, and most traditional material used for bike frames, is steel. It's easy to bend and shape, durable, repairable and inexpensive. It's also heavy, compared to other materials.

One of the lightest, and most popular bike materials— aluminum—became widely used in the 1980s. Although a bit heavier than aluminum, titanium is extremely strong, and became popular in the 1990s as the next "it" material, despite being expensive. This was followed fairly closely by the introduction of carbon fiber, or graphite, in the late 1990s.

It took nearly a decade before the next "must have" material hit the biking scene, in the form of nanocomposites. Easton is playing a pivotal role with next-generation bike materials—their carbon nanotube (CNT) composite made its debut via BMC.

In 2005, BMC introduced its Pro Machine SLC01, whose frame was supplied by Easton. It made its first appearance at the 2005 Tour de France—the Phonak team rode on these bikes. The bike also won a Red Dot Design Award in early 2006. In addition to the SLC01, BMC offers two other bikes with CNT technology: the Team Machine SLT01 and the Cross Machine CX01.

If you want to build your own bike from the ground up, Easton offers a comprehensive range of bike components based on their CNT composite, ranging from handlebars and forks, to the EC90 and EC70 seat posts, as well as the EC70 road stem.

Handlebars include their MonkeyLite MTB Riser Bars, the EC90 and EC70 MTB XC Bars, the EC70 Wing Road Bar, and the Aeroforce Carbon Clip-on Bars. Forks include the EC90 SLX, the EC90 SL, the EC90 Aero, and the EC90 X Cross.

Have you ever wondered how steep that hill you're struggling to climb (or are speeding down) really is? Now you can measure the road's grade with the Bion-CLINO 401 from KOROTEK. About the size of a stopwatch, a MEMS accelerometer provides real-time data regarding incline.

Exercise Equipment

One of the most interesting pieces of exercise equipment I've ever run across is an ideal tool for those of you who love video games. No more passively sitting in front of the TV—now you can be a gamer without being a couch potato (at least prior to the Wii).

I discovered this product several years ago and still think it's pretty ingenious. Called the Exer-Station™, from Interaction Laboratories (formerly called PowerGrid Fitness), the game controller itself (which looks like a handheld game controller), is attached to a post, which in turn is attached to a platform that looks a little bit like a treadmill. Strain gauges provide resistance as you push, pull or turn the controller—my assumption is that this works best with games that don't rely solely on thumb input, like race car driving. So, as you play the game, you actually get a serious workout. The level of resistance is customizable from minimal to nearly 300 pounds.

Extreme Sports

If you mountain bike or snowboard, then you know all about "hang time"—the amount of time that you're up in the air after speeding over a bump of some sort. Now you can actually time it with the HangTimer. About the size of a stopwatch, you clip it onto your ski jacket or shorts and it calculates your "air time" from the moment you leave the ground, until you return (upright or not); it does so via the use of a tri-axis accelerometer. Ruggedized for those not-so-perfect landings, it's also water resistant.

Fishing

Fishermen rejoice. Both MEMS and nanotechnology can help you locate and (hopefully) catch fish better than ever before. Equipment from rods and lures to electronic fish locators are increasingly taking advantage of the latest in new technology. Whether you'll actually catch more fish or not—well, that's another matter entirely.

Fish Finders

Some say that using a fish finder is sort of cheating; that you should be willing to sit in your boat for hours hoping a fish will bite. That's what fishing is all about. Knowing exactly where to cast out a line, because you *know* the area under your boat is just teeming with fish, takes all the fun out of it. Right? I personally think that fish finders are kind of cool, in a cheating sort of way.

Just like GPS is useful for your car, it's useful in fish finders too. Aqua-Vu is a leading manufacturer of electronic underwater viewing systems (otherwise known as fish finders). Their latest products rely on the MEMS magnetic compass from Honeywell to add dead reckoning capability to the GPS signal. When you're out on the lake, if the GPS signal is lost, the MEMS sensors are able to keep track of the distance and direction your boat moves, so once the GPS signal reconnects, it still knows exactly where you are.

Fly Fishing

I haven't come across any regular fishing poles relying on nanomaterials, but there are rods available for those who fly fish. Fly fishing rods are quite different from standard fishing poles in that they're really long (about 9 feet) and super flexible. The whole point is to cast a fly; not a real one, but typically a knot of hair, fur, feathers or other materials meant to look like a fly (or some other insect, depending on the type of fish you're going after).

The art is to make it look like the insect landed on the water's surface, oh-so-briefly, and then is back up in the air flying. Like fishing rods of old, fly fishing rods used to be made of split bamboo, but have since moved to fiberglass, and more recently, carbon fiber or graphite. Nanocomposites made their debut in 2004.

At one point Redington sold the Nano Titanium Quartz (NTiQ) Fly Fishing Rod, but it's no longer available. It used a layer of nanotitanium to enhance graphite, and thus created a stronger rod without compromising flex.

Orvis sells the T3 Fly Fishing Rod, which uses nanoceramic in conjunction with graphite fibers. The end result is a rod that's lighter, tougher and stronger—features that are important for fly fishing. Lighter weight means you won't get tired as fast while casting, and increased toughness means the rod is less prone to cracks; improved strength comes into play when lifting fish.

A third company also sells a line of fly fishing rods based on nanotechnology. But their approach is so unique, that when news of it came out in early 2007, few websites that cover nanotechnology even mentioned it. I'm pretty sure that many simply thought it was a joke, since we're talking carrots here. Really.

CelluComp is leveraging the nanofibers in carrots. Go back to my discussion about composites in Chapter 3 and the use of filler materials, and it starts to make a little more sense. Although I'm still a little skeptical, the use of cellulose as a filler material for nanocomposites is being widely researched. Cellulose is basically the sugar molecules that give wood its strength, and is found in nearly all plants—including carrots. Peel a carrot and you'll see that it does indeed have a string-like texture, unlike peas, for example, that don't (they're mushy rather than stringy).

Called *Curren*™, the material is used in the *Just Cast*™ fly fishing rods. They're available in four lengths and have the same properties as the other fly fishing rods mentioned above.

Lures

Since fish are attracted by motion and color, fishing lures typically rely on bight colors and/or special features meant to reflect sunlight and/or mimic movement to get a fish's attention. In late 2006, ULVAC introduced a new line of lures called STROM, the first known to use nanotechnology, but they're only available in Japan. A special nanocoating results in an iridescent, holographic effect which is said to be more effective than traditional lures with both freshwater and saltwater fish.

Golf

Manufacturers of both MEMS sensors and nanomaterials seem especially fascinated by golf as an end-use. Maybe it's just that golfers are endlessly seeking ways to improve their game, and the most logical place to start is with the equipment.

Golf Balls

NanoDynamics created a lot of buzz when they introduced their NDMX™ golf ball in 2005. It has a hollow metal core (made of proprietary nanoparticles) which is said to yield straighter shots and truer putts. Both the original ball and the new NDLiNX™ are on the United States Golf Association's conforming golf ball list.

Wilson Golf recently introduced several golf balls with its NANO TECH™ core. It's comprised of unknown nanomaterials infused into a soft rubber core. Balls include the Px3 Performance Ball, the Tx4 Tour Ball, the Dx2 Distance Ball, the Lx2 Ladies Ball and the FIFTY 50 Compression Distance Ball. In the case of the latter, it has a new NANO TECH™ core that the company says is 22 percent softer than the original.

Golf Clubs

AccuFLEX offers the Creation 65, Creation 80, Evolution and Evolution Lite shafts for golfers that leverage their proprietary NANOMET technology, a nanometal polymer composite.

Wilson Staff offers two drivers which feature the Nano Tech™ shaft and the Nano Ti™ nano composite crown. Both the Staff Dd5 Nano Ti 460 and Staff Pd5 Nano Ti 400 are on the USGA's list of conforming driver heads.

Yonex offers one of the most extensive lines of golf clubs available (including drivers, fairway woods and irons) whose shafts and crowns both utilize fullerenes. One of their materials, Matrix C60, is a combination of graphite bonded to a fullerene composite to form a lightweight crown. Their second approach, Elastic Ti, is a nanotitanium alloy that results in a shaft that's both highly elastic and incredibly stable.

Product families include the Cyberstar Nanospeed FL driver and the Cyberstar Nanospeed driver, which consist of the following: Cyberstar Nanospeed 420 FL, Cyberstar Nanospeed 460, Cyberstar Nanospeed 460 (LH), Cyberstar Nanov (Ladies), Cyberstar Nanov (LH), Cyberstar Nanov (Version 1), and the Cyberstar Nanov (Version 2). The USGA includes all of these products on their list of conforming driver heads.

Golf Training

MEMS accelerometers, and more recently gyros, are being tapped to help you improve your golf game. One of the first devices to aid in golf swing analysis and training was the Swing-Hat, which looks just like a baseball cap. A MEMS accelerometer embedded in the top monitors swing and then provides audio feedback via an earpiece. It's the least expensive training aid available, at about $100.

Newer products work in a similar manner, but can cost thousands of dollars. The most expensive, which was introduced at the 2006 PGA Merchandise Show, is the Bentley Kinetics K-Vest. It looks like a cross between a harness and a vest, and relies on a MEMS gyroscope for an even greater range of motion sensing.

A slightly different approach comes via the iClub Body Motion System. You can either buy a cap-like module that attaches to the top of the golf club's handle or a vest system similar to the one above. A few years ago another company created a special golf club you could buy called the SmartSwing (it had an accelerometer embedded into the handle itself), but it's no longer available.

Hockey

You wouldn't think that nanotechnology would matter to hockey; but here again, you have a piece of sports equipment in which handling, flexibility and durability is very important. As a result, the materials used over the years in hockey sticks continue to evolve: from wood to fiberglass, then graphite, and now nano-composites.

The longest part of the hockey stick, the shaft, does need some flexibility to transfer the force of slap shots into the puck (the blade actually hits the ice first, a few inches before it hits the puck). To finesse such a shot, a lightweight, flexible shaft is preferred—it's also helpful for overall handling of both the stick and puck during play.

In 2005, Easton introduced their Synergy SL hockey sticks, the first to use a nanocomposite, which allowed for both increased strength and lighter weight. After a bit of refinement, the company now offers a much wider line: Stealth CNT Grip, Stealth CNT, Stealth CNT Grip Intermediate and the Steal CNT Grip JR. The original Synergy line is no longer available.

Montreal Hockey is also using nanotechnology in the shafts of their Nitro line of hockey sticks. Products include the Nitro Lite, Nitro Force, and Nitro Max. They use carbon nanotubes from Bayer MaterialScience.

Hunting

Reliable of Milwaukee (a leading manufacturer of apparel for use in hunting and other outdoor activities), is integrating the SmartSilver™ technology from NanoHorizons in a variety of products that will be available in the fall of 2007. This particular application actually makes a lot of sense. If you hunt frequently and have a special jacket that you wear, it's not likely that it's washed after every outing. As a result, even if you don't think it smells, wildlife can probably catch a whiff of you before you ever see them. If the use of silver nanoparticles can minimize that odor, hunters might just have an advantage here.

Mountain Climbing

A really innovative use of the unique Nanoflex® steel alloy from Sandvik comes courtesy of C.A.M.P. Products, which developed a line a mountain climbing gear with it. This includes the Vector Nanotech and XLC Nanotech crampons (basically, a frame of metal teeth that you attach to the bottom of your boots so you can grip ice), the Corsa Nanotech ice axe and the Nano Wire carabiner (which keeps you attached to your rope).

Personal GPS

Much like navigation systems in cars, which use GPS receivers to pinpoint position and provide route guidance, personal GPS allows you to track where you are—and where you're going—while camping, hiking or doing other outdoor activities. Since GPS on its own isn't 100 percent reliable, adding dead reckoning capability, via MEMS accelerometers, makes it far more accurate.

Two of the leading manufacturers of personal GPS products, Magellan and Garmin, use the MEMS magnetic compass from Honeywell. So as you're hiking, if the GPS signal is lost, the MEMS sensors are able to keep track of the distance and direction you move; once the GPS signal reconnects, it still knows exactly where you are (well, within a foot or two).

Protective Gear

There's a lot of protective gear used in sports, much of which is plastic, so it would make sense that nanomaterials might come into play at some point. In the meantime, nanosilver certainly is; as is nanometal. The one technology that's making quite an impact (literally) is shear thickening fluid and similar approaches discussed in Chapter 9.

Core Protection/Mouth Guards

Shock Doctor is a leading supplier of mouth guards and other core protective gear for use in football, hockey, lacrosse and other sports. In early 2007, the company announced that it was incorporating SmartSilver™ from NanoHorizons into many of their products. They'll be available in the fall of 2007.

Face Guards

Sandvik, who manufactures a unique nanometal found in electric shavers, has also found application of their product in sports masks that rely on metal grids to guard the face—like those worn by hockey players and baseball catchers.

Gloves

Sells, who makes protective equipment for soccer players, makes special gloves for soccer goalkeepers that have a strip of the d3o material across the knuckles to better protect their hands during play. They became available in 2006.

Reusch created special gloves for snowboarders using the d3o material to protect the palm of the hand, which makes sense given the need to grip the board, touching down to turn, as well as the instinct to cushion a fall with your hand.

In early 2007, JPMS introduced several gloves for motorcycle racers which also feature the d3o material on the knuckle area. This doesn't make quite as much sense to me as its use in soccer or snowboarding gloves, but then, I don't watch motorcycle racing enough to know what kind of hand protection they really need.

Head Protection

RibCap uses the technology from d3o for use in a line of "flexible helmets" for sports such as snowboarding. They actually look like any other knitted wool cap, except that sections of them are made from d3o's unique material. So if you fall and hit your head, you'll have some impact protection, even though it doesn't look like you're wearing a helmet. Making a fashion statement on the slopes is a big deal, and the RibCap does this—while protecting you at the same time. I should point out (as the company does) that these caps don't offer full head protection like a helmet does; but they are a better alternative to wearing nothing. Similar caps/beanies will be available from both Ignite and Quicksilver in time for winter 2007/2008.

For serious head protection, and I'm talking football here, you might be interested in the Sideline Response System™ from the leading supplier of sports equipment, Riddell, who makes use of the Head Impact Telemetry™ technology developed by Simbex. MEMS accelerometers are embedded into the football helmet itself, which, along with other electronics, sends the data captured to a system located on the sidelines, which records it for analysis. It can provide a warning if any particular impact seems especially dangerous; that is, likely to result in real injury. It's been in use in college football since 2005.

Running/Walking

Because MEMS accelerometers monitor motion, they're a great way to measure the speed or distance you travel while walking or running. Their use continues to expand from pedometers you clip on your pants, to pods you attach to your shoes (which wirelessly transmits data to a special watch you wear)—even some cell phones have a pedometer function!

Part of the reason for the growing popularity of pedometers is the challenge to walk 10,000 steps per day. Even increasing the number of steps you walk each day by 2,000 can be beneficial to your health. Here are three examples of some products:

- Garmin's Forerunner 305 gives you the option to use GPS or a foot pod, the latter of which relies on two accelerometers to measure each stride to provide running speed and distance information. The data is wirelessly sent to the Forerunner wrist watch.

- Nike's unique Nike+iPod system allows a special running shoe to wirelessly transmit speed and distance data to your iPod Nano. The MEMS accelerometer is actually sold separately in the Sport Kit, it's then inserted into a special pocket of the shoe. An enterprising company has come up with a small pouch that allows you to use the sensor from the Sport Kit with any running shoe.

- Omron's HJ-7201TC is their newest pedometer to rely on a MEMS accelerometer to keep track of the number of steps you walk.
- Teltronic's ikcal measures calorie burning (via physical activity) compared to food consumption and determines whether a person is getting a sufficient amount of exercise. It relies on a tri-axis accelerometer from VTI Technologies.

Scuba Diving

One of the first consumer-oriented applications of MEMS pressures sensors was in SCUBA gear. In recent years they've expanded from use in the tank equipment (to monitor air pressure) to integration into the mask itself, as well as dive computers. This makes sense, since MEMS pressure sensors are found in most sports watches with a barometer function.

Dive computers, which look like wrist watches, measure the depth and time of the dive, as well as provide information such as water temperature, amount of air left and many other pieces of data pertinent to diving. Key to depth measurement is a pressure sensor. Some of the newest models also incorporate an electronic compass. It's not known if they're relying on the same technology as those found in personal GPS systems, but since MEMS sensors are so tiny, it's certainly a possibility.

Skiing

From the skis themselves to the clothes you wear while swooshing down the slopes, nanotechnology is making a real difference for skiers. If you haven't already, take a look at the "Protective Gear" section above (there's a cool knit cap available that doubles as a helmet).

Ski Wax

The product that really created a lot of buzz for nanotechnology as a whole is Nanogate's Cerax Nanowax. Despite the name, it's not a wax, it's actually a polymer.

Skiers wax their skis so that they either grip the snow better (a property important for cross-country skiing), or glide better (a property important for downhill skiing). Ski wax is quite an art—much depends on the temperature (is it above or below freezing), as well as what kind of snow it is—heavy, wet snow or fluffy, dry powder. For gliding, the whole point is to find just the right balance of water between the snow and the ski—too much results in suction, while not enough causes friction.

Formulated at the nanoscale, Nanowax allows for both high gliding and good sticking, depending on the temperature. The line includes Uni Wax (a universal product), AS WET (for wet snow), AS DRY (for dry snow) and RACE 1, 2 and 3. They're useful for both skis and snowboards.

Skis

Atomic sells the only line of skis so far which benefit from the use of nanomaterials. Their Izor skis rely on a nano silicon oxide and carbon fiber in a special frame, which is shaped sort of like a "U" and attached to a flat ski. The curved part is placed at the tip and the open end is at the tail. This makes the skis extremely light, and allows them to "turn effortlessly with excellent edge grip, support, and control," and thus require little energy to ride. Four Izor skis are available, the 9:7m, the 7:5m, the 5:3m, and the 3:1m.

Ski Clothes

If you've watched an alpine ski event (where skiers race down a course lined with gates they inevitably run over as they go around them), you might wonder how bruised they get from hitting them. Its obvious those gate poles are flexible, but that still has to hurt.

In Chapter 9 I talked about the various kinds of "liquid armor" being developed, a material that is typically soft and flexible, but becomes hard upon impact. One of the first applications of this technology was actually on TV for the world to see at the 2006 Olympics in Torino. In late 2005, Spyder created racing suits for the US and Canadian alpine ski teams, which they wore during the slalom and giant slalom events. They used the d3o technology on the shins, forearms and elbows to protect the racers against collisions with the race gates. Spyder launched a line of race suits with the technology in late 2006 for sale to the general public.

Along those lines, Schöffel sells the Protector S2 High-Tech Protector ski jacket (and pants) that include removable elbow and shoulder pads made of the d3o material. Or, you could buy the fleece vest from Kjus, which uses d3o material as a detachable back protector. An alternative is to wear thermal underwear with the material placed on the elbows and knees, like Sessions has with their Thermatics d3o Crew and Pant.

Snowboarding

Between the HangTimer and the RibCap, snowboarders might feel like MEMS and nanotechnology has their sport well covered, but there's one more product to talk about: the snowboard itself. Yonex, who's best known for badminton and tennis racquets, also sells a snowboard, which relies on fullerenes. The Air Carbon Tube Smooth was specifically designed for use on half-pipes and jump ramps; the fullerenes increase both the board's strength and bouncing power.

Tennis

One of the most innovative pieces of sports equipment to make use of nanomaterials was the Wilson Double Core tennis balls, which made their debut in early 2001. To understand what a big deal it was, it would probably help to understand the construction of tennis balls themselves.

Tennis balls are comprised of an inner core and an outer layer of fabric. Back in the earliest days of tennis, the balls were made with a variety of materials, including hair and leather. One of the most popular was strips of wool wrapped around a cork core, held together with string and then covered with cloth. The use of vulcanized rubber emerged about 100 years ago as a core material, and remains the standard today.

There are actually two types of tennis balls: pressurized and non-pressurized. Pressurized balls have, logically enough, pressurized air in the core. It makes sense then that they lose pressure over time and become unplayable; typically within two weeks after being taken out of the can. Non-pressurized tennis balls have a thicker rubber core and wear out when the outer covering does. Supposedly you can't tell the difference, but pro players prefer to use pressurized balls.

What made the Wilson Double Core tennis balls so unique is that they were a pressurized ball that lasted twice as long. They did so by using a thin layer of nanoclay composite to coat the core. This highly efficient barrier prevented the air from dissipating as quickly. Unfortunately, the balls are no longer being made. Given the number of tennis balls sold on a yearly basis, perhaps they were too efficient. It is an interesting observation considering that nanomaterials haven't been used in tennis balls since—most of the focus has turned to the racquets.

Manufacturers are continually trying to create the ultimate tennis racquet: one that's both ultra-strong and ultra-light, with lower elasticity, higher torsional stability and optimal power for greater ball speed and control. Nanomaterials appear to be the answer. But if you think that only carbon nanotubes can do that, think again. In addition to carbon nanotubes, nanoparticles of silicon dioxide and titanium are also being used—as well as aerogels. Read on.

In late 2001, Babolat made waves by introducing the first tennis racquet leveraging carbon nanotubes. But questions were raised as to whether it was simply a marketing ploy, since the amount of nanomaterial actually used was pretty minimal. In the end, it doesn't matter anymore, since the company now offers tennis racquets that leverage a graphite/carbon nanotube composite in both the head and shaft: the NS Tour and NS Drive.

Dunlop introduced a new line of tennis racquets leveraging aerogels in early 2007. It actually makes sense, given the fact that aerogels are the lightest material on earth, with a strength that's 4,000 times its weight. Dunlop is combining aerogel with their Multi-Filament Technology, which results in a stiffer top of the frame; this minimizes movement and creates more power. At the bottom of the racquet head, aerogel provides torsional stability. Racquets available include the Dunlop Aerogel 2Hundred, 3Hundred, 5Hundred, and 5Hundred Tour.

HEAD offers the Nano Titanium series of tennis racquets, which are a "composite weave of ultra-strong titanium and ultra-light graphite fibers for maximum weight reduction, optimal stiffness, and power." Racquets in the series include the Ti.S6, Ti.S4, Ti.S2, Ti.S1, Ti.Fire, Ti.Heat, and Ti.Ice.

In late 2006, HEAD introduced a brand new series called Metallix, which combines carbon fibers and nanometal from PowerMetal Technologies to create a "nanocrystalline reinforcement layer to stiffen the shaft of the racquets." Two racquets are currently available: the Metallix 6 and Metallix 10.

Wilson offers the n1Force Tennis Racquet, which uses their nCode technology. Here, "nano-sized silicon dioxide crystals permeate the voids between the carbon fibers." The result is a racquet that's "2x stronger, 2x more stable, and up to 22 percent more powerful." In late 2006, Wilson ran ads for its nCode tennis racquet starring Roger Federer.

Wilson's newest racquet technology, [K]Factor, takes their nCode technology a step further by bonding carbon black, graphite and silicon dioxide at the nanoscale for a denser, stronger, more stable racquet. They call the new material [K]arophite Black. Roger Federer won the Australian Open in early 2007 playing with the [K]Six racquet.

Yonex uses Elastic Ti, a nanoscale alloy of titanium, which "has 44 percent lower elasticity and 8 percent higher strength" compared to titanium alloys. Racquets featuring Elastic Ti "will snap-back quicker to give higher repulsion power" for improved stability. This basically results in greater ball speed and control of the racquet. The racquets also use Matrix C60, which combines fullerenes with carbon fibers. Tennis racquets include the RQS-11, the NSRQ-8, the NSRQ-7, and the NSRQ-5.

Logic will get you from A to B. Imagination will take you everywhere.

—*Albert Einstein*

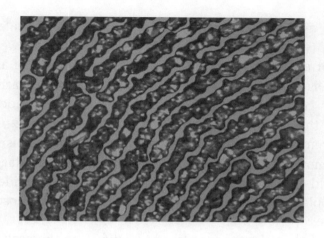

11 • HEALTHCARE/MEDICINE

MEMS and nanotechnology are both frequently referred to as having a revolutionary impact on all sorts of different products and markets. But the description is perhaps best applied to medicine, where the use of these technologies truly is profound. Most of the innovations available today are products used by doctors, nurses, researchers and other medical professionals. However, there are a growing number of healthcare products readily available to consumers (i.e. in your local pharmacy or drug store), that rely on MEMS or nanotechnology in some way.

Medicine is an attractive market for nano/MEMS suppliers for two key reasons: a rapidly aging population and increased incidence of obesity worldwide. In 2006, almost 500 million people worldwide were older than 65. Just 25 years from now, that total will double to 1 billion[13] people, and account for 12.5 percent of the world's population. This alone will put serious economic strain on countries worldwide, most notably in terms of healthcare.

As for as the incidence of obesity; it's reaching crisis levels. As of 2005, two-thirds of all adults in the United States were overweight or obese. In terms of obesity alone, one-third of all adults over the age of 20 fall into this category[14]. Even more alarming are statistics concerning children. Seventeen percent of adolescents between the ages of 12–19 are overweight, and nearly 20 percent of children younger than 11 are overweight[15]. And this isn't just a U.S. phenomenon. The global numbers for obesity are staggering— the World Health Organization estimates that, worldwide, one in four people are now overweight and one-quarter of those people are obese[16].

Both of these issues are already manifesting themselves in an increased number of cardiovascular and diabetes-related issues. More than 25 million US adults have heart disease[17], and at least 16 million live with diabetes[18]; those are just the diagnosed cases.

The good news is that MEMS and nanomaterials are already providing subtle, but tangible improvements in preventative care, diagnosis, treatment and patient outcomes (or the result of treatment). Even more exciting are the MEMS devices and nanotechnology-based approaches in the development pipeline anticipated to come to market over the next five years and beyond.

This is such a fascinating area, that I'm going to split the chapter into two parts. In Part 1, I'll talk about the kind of products that you can find in the healthcare aisle of most stores; Part 2 will discuss how MEMS and nanotechnology are changing the tools and equipment used by those within the medical community. Either way, you're the one who ultimately benefits from the incredible advances being made.

PART 1 – HEALTHCARE

Asthma

Asthma is a modern day issue that affects tens of millions of people worldwide. In the United States alone, at least 16 million adults[19] and 7 million children[20] have asthma, an inflammatory disease of the lungs which makes breathing difficult. Exercise, obesity, stress and others factors can trigger asthma attacks; it is now the most common chronic childhood disease. While the exact cause isn't entirely understood, it appears to be an effect of industrialization. Some point to increased pollution and lower air quality, as well as second-hand smoke; others think it's because kids spend too much time indoors. It's even been suggested that dust mites, cat dander, cockroaches and mold play roles, but no one really knows.

Asthma attacks are controlled by medicine administered with devices called inhalers, the most common of which is a metered dose inhaler (MDI). It provides a certain number of doses, which range from 60 to 240 puffs (or inhalations) per unit. Asthma severity is tracked by the number of puffs of medication needed on a daily basis.

The best way to administer asthma medicine is when you first begin to inhale. However, MDIs tend to be activated during emergency situations—the anxiety caused from not being able to breathe well means that the MDI could be triggered when the lungs are full or when the person is exhaling. This not only wastes medicine, but also prolongs the amount of time it takes for the medicine to get into the lungs and start working.

Many MDIs use pressure sensors to detect where an individual is in the breathing cycle and to release the medication at the appropriate time to optimize drug delivery. In addition, most nozzles in MDIs today are micromachined, which results in an incredibly precise array of holes. This means that the spray droplets are finer and more uniform, and thus better targeted into the lungs. The bottom line is that the medicine works more effectively, and less is wasted.

One of the most advanced MDIs on the market today is the Respimat® Soft Mist™ Inhaler from Boehringer Ingelheim. It relies on a unique nozzle structure (called the Uniblock) developed by Steag microParts, whom Boehringer Ingelheim acquired.

Blood Pressure

We live in an increasingly stressful world, and it shows. About 30 percent of US adults have hypertension[21] (high blood pressure), so many of you may have an electronic blood pressure monitor at home. If you do, you might be benefiting from a MEMS pressure sensor. Omron is a leading manufacturer of not only blood pressure monitoring equipment (for use by both consumers and medical professionals), but the MEMS pressure sensor inside them. These tiny sensors not only provide more precise readings, but they've also allowed for the development of products such as blood pressure monitors that just clip onto the end of your finger.

Contact Lenses

At the American Chemical Society's national meeting in 2005, chemists from both Ciba Vision and Bausch & Lomb revealed that they use both micro and nanoscale particles of titanium dioxide, iron oxide and barium sulfate, as well as nanoscale films, to create their colored contact lenses[22]. However, after reading Chapter 3, we now know that many pigments today are produced at the nanoscale, so this shouldn't come as a surprise. When colored lenses first appeared on the market, it was pretty obvious when someone wore such lenses. Today's colored contact lenses certainly look much more realistic.

Feminine Hygiene

Ladies (and men) take note: the next time you send your significant other to the store (or you get sent) on that unbearable errand of purchasing feminine hygiene pads, you can make sure to purchase a product that supports nanotechnology and the environment at the same time. The Flushaway™ brand uses nanofilms in the pad and liner. The product works the same as others on the market, but the use of nanoscale materials results in a biodegradable product that starts to break down as soon as you flush it (yes, it's actually flushable).

First Aid

With all of the focus on the use of silver as an antimicrobial, it was only a matter of time before bandages hopped on board. Actually, it turns out they were one of the first. Back in 2004, Beiersdorf launched their CURAD® Silver bandages, which reduce bacterial growth in the dressing for 24 hours. It looks and is applied like any other traditional bandage, but there's no need for a topical antibacterial cream, since silver ions are infused within the bandage pad itself. Note the use of ions here—not nanoparticles. The reason I point this out is because I did see a number references to the product stating the use of nanoparticles, which as we've learned, is incorrect.

Analgesic

As many of you are probably aware, you don't have to be an athlete or exercise warrior to suffer from aches and pains; mowing the lawn or shoveling the snow is sometimes enough. There are a number of analgesic creams on the market that help to ease sore muscles and one now appears to use nanotechnology. Flex-Power Joint & Muscle Pain Relief is said to use a "nanotech delivery system" so that the ingredients penetrate more deeply into the skin, making the product more effective.

However, the FLEX-SOME™ technology is actually based on the use of "microscopic lipid spheres," or liposomes. As I discussed in Chapter 8, liposomes are a nanoscale approach to encapsulating ingredients, but it is not necessarily nanotechnology. Does the differentiation ultimately matter? To some, yes; to others, probably not. The bottom line is that we're talking about a product that uses an advanced technology which allows ingredients to better penetrate the skin, so that they can provide a tangible effect; in this case, reduce muscle soreness.

Hearing Aids

It used to be that the elderly were the most likely to need a hearing aid, but it's clear that people are experiencing hearing loss at a much younger age. The numbers vary, but up to 50 percent of high-school and college students now suffer from a greater level of noise-induced hearing loss than their parents. In fact, if that percentage holds true, hearing loss amongst youth is more on par with what one would generally expect for a person in their seventies. Many are pointing their fingers at the use of portable music players, and even cell phones.

More than 36 million adults have hearing trouble[23], which is up from 28 million just five years ago. However, only 20 percent of people who need hearing aids actually wear one[24]. Why the resistance? The stigma of wearing a visible hearing aid is the primary reason, although the development of hearing aids that hide inside the ear has helped. The reluctance appears to be disappearing recently, and some attribute that to the popularity of Bluetooth headsets used with cell phones. But let's face it, hearing aids can be very expensive, and often don't work well.

Many of today's hearing aids now use MEMS microphones, which offer vastly improved quality over older microphone technologies. In addition, Siemens recently introduced an ultra-thin, anti-adhesive coating (using nanoparticles) for use on their newest behind-the-ear (BTE) hearing aids. The nanocoating repels water and sweat, thus reducing moisture-related failures and repairs.

Mobility

Loss of mobility generally results in a real (or perceived) loss of independence, a very emotionally difficult thing to deal with, no matter what age you are.

Innovative Neurotronics developed the WalkAid® system, a device meant to improve the gait of patients who have a lack of ankle dorsiflexion, due to spinal cord damage, which is called Foot Drop. In other words, they have trouble lifting their foot, making it difficult to walk correctly. The device restores functionality by mimicking and recreating nerve-to-nerve responses via electrical stimulation; a MEMS accelerometer monitors leg and foot movements. About the size of a deck of cards, it's worn on the leg, just below the knee.

In terms of prosthetics, real advances are being made. One of the most successful prosthetics is the C-Leg from Otto Bock Healthcare, which uses strain gauges to enhance its movement in response to the wearer. The recent reduction in the price of MEMS gyro sensors and accelerometers may make an even more significant difference here. A new prosthetic from Ossur North America, the Proprio Foot, is a great example. It uses a gyro sensor to help articulate the ankle, resulting in a more natural foot movement while walking.

There was considerable buzz in late 2001 when Dean Kaman unveiled the Segway® Personal Transporter. What many probably don't realize is that it had a precursor: the INDEPENDENCE® iBOT® Mobility System, one of the most unique wheelchairs ever developed.

At the core of the iBOT Mobility System is its iBALANCE® Technology, which also relies on multiple MEMS gyro sensors and accelerometers to provide balance. And how is balance important in a wheelchair? The iBOT Mobility System can lift its user to a standing height, balancing on just two wheels, so that the person in the wheelchair can interact with others face-to-face. The importance of this cannot be emphasized enough.

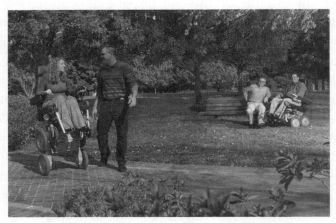

Photo courtesy of Independence Technology LLC

It took several years to gain FDA approval, partly because it seemed as though the FDA couldn't believe that the chair worked the way it did. I recall news stories at the time about the kinds of tests conducted, and I can understand the FDA's incredulity. This was prior to the unveiling of the Segway Personal Transporter, so nothing like it had ever been seen before. To ease concerns about safety, the chair has "triple redundant back-up systems," meaning it contains three identical sets of the MEMS gyro/accelerometer sensor cluster that makes it work.

The iBOT Mobility System works in both four- and two-wheel mode. It can roll smoothly over uneven terrain, climb up and over obstacles such as stairs or high curbs, and, as mentioned, lift its user to a standing height. This wheelchair not only makes interaction with other people more normal, but things we take for granted, like grocery shopping or taking dishes out of the cupboard at home, is also much easier.

Scales

I can't think of too many people who don't have a scale in their bathroom. If yours is electronic, more likely than not, MEMS strain gauges from Measurement Specialties are what helps to determine your weight.

Thermometers

It's been nearly a decade now since MEMS transformed the way we take our temperature. Forget the mercury-based thermometer you had to hold under your tongue, many parents today use a thermometer placed in the ear for just a moment. Most ear thermometers now use a thermopile for instant, non-contact temperature measurement. When I say non-contact, I mean that the sensor itself doesn't contact the ear (although the thermometer housing does). Yes, this is the same kind of sensor that's found in your hair dryer and microwave.

PART 2 – MEDICINE

I'm sure you've seen a lot of talk in the press about "nanobots" and how they'll someday wander through our bodies helping to fix whatever is ailing us. I cringe a little bit at the use of the term, because while it refers to an inanimate object, news accounts make it sound like a sentient, living creature. In reality, the concept is far less scary than you might think. The bottom line is that these are basically smart systems—such as implantable sensors and time-release drug delivery structures. I suppose knowing that takes the fun out of the more fantastic, futuristic scenario of tiny walking, talking robots scurrying around making you well, but it also puts the concept into a more realistic perspective. Besides, this isn't the stuff of tomorrow as many indicate—they're already in use today.

For the rest of this chapter, we'll see how MEMS and nanotechnology are changing the tools used by healthcare professionals. I'll discuss two key areas where much of the product development efforts are focused, as well as the impact of nano/MEMS on diagnostic tools, equipment and materials, infection control and pharmaceuticals.

Areas of Focus

An aging population that's increasingly overweight presents some very real issues that the medical community is working hard to address: more people with heart disease and diabetes. It's no wonder that many firms who are developing MEMS devices and working with nanomaterials are focusing their efforts on what is clearly two of the biggest commercial opportunities.

Cardiology

The number of cardiovascular procedures in the United States alone increased at a blistering pace over the past two decades—up nearly 400 percent. More than 2 million people now undergo angioplasty or have a stent, pacemaker or defibrillator implanted.

Angioplasty (also called Balloon Angioplasty, or Percutaneous Transluminal Coronary Angioplasty—PTCA) is a procedure to open clogged arteries by inserting a tiny balloon into the blocked area to open the vessel. Here's how it's done:

A very thin, stainless steel wire, called a guidewire, is used as a positioning tool for a catheter. The guidewire is typically inserted into the body through an incision made to the main artery in the upper thigh of the patient. The guidewire is then advanced up into the coronary arteries to the blockage area. Once positioned, a hollow catheter is placed over the guidewire and pushed along until the tip of the catheter reaches the blockage. A collapsed balloon at the tip of the catheter is then inflated, compressing the plaque build-up against the artery wall. This enlarges the opening of the vessel and allows for better blood flow to the heart.

Positioning of the guidewire and catheter used to depend entirely on the skill and experience of the physician. However, the integration of MEMS sensors makes the guidewires and catheters more intelligent, and thus the physician can place them with greater accuracy. RADI Medical Systems makes a catheter, the PressureWire®5, which not only measures pressure, but temperature and blood flow as well.

In many cases, during an angioplasty, a stent (a tiny, metal, scaffolding-like device) is placed into the newly opened artery to keep it open. Amongst other challenges, the stent must be easily compressed onto the balloon catheter (which delivers it), adhere to the catheter so that it is not lost during the placement process and be able to adequately open the vessel. If that's not enough, stents must also have enough structural strength to hold the vessel walls open for years in tough conditions; it must resist corrosion, be able to withstand constant flexing and stay in place.

Stents are fabricated out of a stainless steel tube that is laser micromachined in intricate patterns that make them as flexible as possible, while maintaining the rigidity necessary to keep from closing. Laser micromachining, as a process, is a bit of a gray area as it pertains to MEMS. Some consider the process a MEMS manufacturing technique (since you're ultimately creating a three-dimensional object that performs a mechanical function), whereas others do not. However, there are some stents in development that are specifically described to as MEMS devices.

Do you know anyone who has a pacemaker or a defibrillator? These two devices help correct how a patient's heart functions. What helps them do that today is a MEMS accelerometer.

Defibrillators control heart rhythm. Some people's hearts beat dangerously fast (called ventricular tachycardia), whereas others beat so chaotically (ventricular fibrillation), that rather than beating, they almost quiver. Both conditions can lead to cardiac arrest or a heart attack. An implantable cardioverter-defibrillator (ICD) senses these irregular conditions and provides electrical shocks to restore a normal heart rhythm.

Pacemakers regulate heart beat. Some people's hearts beat too slowly (called bradycardia). This may be due to the natural aging process, the result of a heart attack (and the muscle is damaged), or a genetic condition. A pacemaker mimics the heart by generating electrical impulses to maintain a proper heart beat. In the past, pacemakers worked at a fixed rate. Today's pacemakers are increasingly sophisticated; for example, they can detect if you're exercising and adjust your heart rate accordingly.

The U.S. Food and Drug Administration recently opened the door to a whole new frontier for the use of MEMS sensing in medicine: implantable sensors. The first applications focus on the aorta, the largest artery in your body.

In late 2005, CardioMEMS received FDA approval for their EndoSure™ AAA Wireless Pressure Measurement System, which is implanted at the same time a patient has a stent-graft inserted during an endovascular aortic repair (EVAR). In this case, the aorta weakens and balloons in the abdominal area. Once in place, doctors monitor the patient's condition by placing an antenna on the patient's abdomen; this activates the sensor and creates a waveform on a monitor so the doctor can interpret the data.

In early 2007, CardioMEMS received FDA clearance for a second application: thoracic aortic aneurysm (TAA) repair. In this case, the aorta weakens and balloons in the chest area. The sensor then provides real-time information about pressure, heart rate and cardiac output.

Diabetes

In just the past 20 years, the number of people worldwide with diabetes increased eight-fold, to hundreds of millions. In the United States, more than 20 million people (roughly 7 percent of the population), has diabetes[25]. Between Type I and Type II diabetes, most people have Type II, and many point to the proliferation of obesity as the primary reason for the increase in this type of diabetes.

With Type I diabetes, the pancreas no longer makes insulin, whereas with Type II, either not enough insulin is produced, or what is produced doesn't work properly. In both instances, blood glucose levels need to be monitored so that those with Type I diabetes can determine how much insulin to inject, and those with Type II diabetes can keep their insulin levels steady.

One of the most difficult aspects of the disease is the need to continually monitor blood glucose levels. This is accomplished by taking blood samples, typically from the finger, multiple times daily. Many diabetics simply do not do this as frequently as they should due to the pain of needle sticks.

Much of the innovation in MEMS is focused on making the management of diabetes easier. They range from finer needles (so there's less pain), to fully implantable systems that can monitor blood glucose and automatically delivery insulin when needed. The "holy grail" is the development of an implantable solution for the long-term monitoring of blood glucose and automatic insulin of delivery; basically, an artificial pancreas.

Debiotech took a step in that direction in early 2006 with the introduction of the Nanopump™, one of the smallest insulin pumps on the market. Although not fully implantable, the device delivers insulin subcutaneously (just under the skin) for about 7 days before it needs to be replaced.

Diagnostic Tools

Quickly, efficiently and cost-effectively determining a patient's condition is often critical to accurate, timely treatment. Almost all diagnostic tests fall into four basic categories: those that take measurements (i.e. heart rate, lung function and vision), those that take something out of the body to study (such as blood or urine), those that look at the body (i.e. x-ray and ultrasound) and those that look inside the body (endoscopes).

Both MEMS and nanomaterials are resulting in both the enhancement of existing imaging technologies, and the creation of new ones, such as new ultrasound devices and imaging dyes; but these are still in development. In the meantime, let's take a look at how the other diagnostic categories are benefiting.

Measurements

Blood pressure measurement is one of the most basic diagnostic tools, and can be done in one of several ways: via manual cuffs (sphygmomanometers), automatic or continual non-invasive devices (wrist cuffs or inserting one's finger into a portable device) and invasive arterial monitoring (as part of an IV line).

Continuous monitoring of blood pressure is critical during and after surgery. In this case, disposable pressure sensors are used in conjunction with IV lines to monitor blood pressure during surgery and recovery. The advantage of this system is that blood pressure is constantly monitored beat-by-beat, and a waveform (a graph of pressure against time) can be displayed. This type of blood pressure monitoring is generally reserved for critically ill patients where rapid variations in blood pressure are anticipated.

Specimens

Specimens such as blood or urine are necessary to test for specific things that can point out what's wrong (or what's not), i.e. is your liver functioning properly, are you losing blood, are you in shock, etc. Such tests are a necessity in the emergency room, and both during and after surgery. They're also used as a basic diagnostic tool in doctors' offices.

STAT tests are required by critical care physicians in areas such as emergency rooms, intensive care/critical care units and surgical suites, because of the time sensitive nature of their treatment. In the past, tests sent to the hospital's central laboratory could take hours, a delay which certainly affected patient treatment in urgent situations. As a result, STAT laboratories were established to reduce this time delay, but the test costs were significantly higher.

Lab-on-a-chip has truly revolutionized the way hospitals handle many diagnostic tests. The result is a new approach to patient diagnosis and monitoring, and even better, the way patients are managed, or taken care of.

Today's point-of-care (POC) diagnostics, such as the i-STAT® system, allows a medical professional to draw a few drops of blood from the patient, place the specimen in a chip, insert the chip into the reader and get results back in as little as two minutes. Most readers are about the size of a cordless phone and the chips themselves are about the size of the compact flash card that you use in your digital camera.

If you watch TV medical shows, you might hear the emergency room "doctors" yelling out the need for a "CBC Chem 7" or something along those lines as a patient is dramatically rolled into the emergency room. Those tests are real.

CBC is short for complete blood count, and includes measurements like hematocrit, which can indicate blood loss. Blood chemistries such as glucose are important, because the patient might be diabetic. Measuring things like blood gases and electrolytes can determine if the patient is in shock, and of course, there are various tests to determine liver and kidney functions. All can affect diagnosis and/or treatment choice, as well as rule out specific conditions, or point to the need for more specific tests.

Did you know that more than 6 million people in the U.S. go to the emergency room for chest pain[26]? In some instances it can take up to 24 hours to determine whether the patient is having a heart attack or not because of the tests that need to be repeated. But that's changing.

During a heart attack, certain proteins are released from the damaged heart muscle into the bloodstream. These proteins vary in concentration and consist of CK-MB, troponin I and myoglobin. Myoglobin is the earliest of the markers to be detected and the first to leave the body. Both CK-MB and troponin I are later markers, but they stay in the body longer and are more specific to cardiac damage from a heart attack.

Biosite Diagnostics was the first to develop a lab-on-a-chip test to specifically detect these proteins, but others are catching up and offering these tests as well. The i-STAT system can detect cardiac markers in just five minutes. That can make a profound difference in patient care.

But it goes beyond simple blood tests. The DNA-based lab-on-a-chip devices developed for life science research have basically been combined with the rapid results capability of point-of-care diagnostics, which has opened up a whole new market. I refer to this as clinical diagnostics. These are tests where time isn't necessarily of the essence; you don't need the results in minutes, but getting a diagnosis within a few days (rather than a few weeks) could make a real difference. This is where we're seeing the development of lab-on-a-chip to detect viruses and bacteria like bird flu and E. coli, and even cancer. For example, Combimatrix has a lab-on-a-chip test that allows pathologists to discriminate between malignant melanoma and benign moles.

One application of such tests is for an emerging area called personalized medicine; the ability to create drugs for a particular condition, but tailored to specific genetics. Not everyone responds in the same way to medicine, so the point is to create medicines that will work as efficiently as possible—for *you*. It's not as far-fetched as you might think.

IPSOGEN sells chips that not only allow for the profiling of cancer (with a specific focus on breast cancer), but for the development of cancer drugs. By being able to specifically identify the tumor type (and there are many, each of which has a different prognosis, or outcome), treatments can be better tailored to each patient. Eventually, this kind of information will allow researchers to develop drugs specific to each class of tumor, ultimately resulting in better chances of treatment success—and hopefully with fewer side effects.

Speaking of blood tests, I'm sure most of you have had a health-care professional draw several vials of blood from your arm to run all sorts of tests, or insert an IV line into a vein in the back of your hand. Many of those people are very, very good; they find the vein and get the needle or catheter in before you can blink. I've personally experienced one or two who, well, let's just say their inability to get the needle into the vein was such that I'd never let them get close to me (or my veins) ever again. But there's a fascinating new technology that may very well make such bad experiences a thing of the past.

The VeinViewer by Luminetx™ uses infrared light to illuminate veins just below the skin. The system then uses the DLP® from Texas Instruments to basically project an image of the veins on the skin's surface. The end result is a "map" of the veins, so healthcare professionals know *exactly* where your veins are.

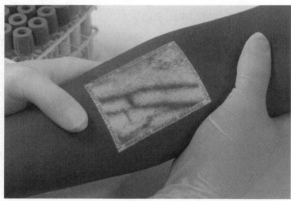

Creating an image of the arm's veins. © *2006 Luminetx Technologies Corporation.*

Endoscopes

Endoscopes, which are thin, flexible tubes that allow doctors to see into the body, have done wonders for the ability to diagnose certain illnesses. Current endoscopes rely on MEMS pressure sensors to measure pressure in the stomach or other organs in which the endoscope is inserted. As with other areas in which MEMS and nanotechnology are playing a role, endoscopy is now starting to evolve as well.

One device that perhaps best embodies the "nanobots" concept is the diagnostic pill. Rather than relying on a tube inserted into the gastrointestinal tract (which can only go so far), patients can now swallow a "pill" full of various sensors, lights and tiny cameras, which takes pictures and other measurements as it passes through the entire GI system. Several companies now offer such devices for the diagnosis of a variety of conditions.

The SmartPill GI Monitoring System assesses gastro motility in the intestinal tract—basically, digestive problems. You swallow the SmartPill pH.p capsule, and go about your daily business.

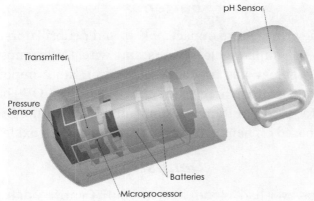

Close-up of a diagnostic pill. Diagram courtesy of SmartPill Corporation.

As the "pill" works its way through the digestive tract, MEMS pressure and temperature sensors, as well as a pH sensor, transmits data to an external receiver that the patient wears. When the pill passes from the body, the patient returns the receiver to the physician so they can assess the data.

The SmartPill is by no means the only such product that does this—imaging of the small intestine has truly been transformed. Given Imaging received FDA approval of their PillCam™ back in 2001; uses include the detection of abnormalities, disorders and injuries such as Crohn's Disease, as well as both benign and malignant tumors. The EndoCapsule from Olympus Medical Systems detects things like bleeding.

Equipment/Materials

There's a lot of equipment and materials used by healthcare professionals that you come in direct contact with, but you've probably never given a second thought to how they work. Maybe you'll look at some a little bit differently next time you use them.

Batteries

With the growing use of pacemakers and defibrillators, and the emergence of implantable sensors and wireless diagnostic pills, battery technology has probably never been more important. In early 2007, Greatbatch revealed that its nanoSVO™ battery is qualified for incorporation into implantable medical devices. The battery is based on nanoparticles of silver vanadium oxide.

Dentistry

Have you ever had a tooth knocked out? Dentistry dates back to the ancient Egyptians—and some of the first known dental implants were actually used by the Mayans[27]. A dental implant is a replacement for an entire tooth structure; it's basically a titanium screw fixed into the bone your teeth are attached to. Bone then grows on its surface to fully integrate it into the jaw. A crown, bridge or dental prosthesis is then attached to the implant. In the case of the ancient Mayans, they used shells as both the implant and the tooth. Fast-forward about two thousand years and nano-materials are coming into play.

BoneGen-TR from BioLok International is a time-release, nanocomposite of calcium sulfate to promote bone attachment. It can be used in a wide array of dental procedures, including bone regeneration and augmentation, as well as a soft-tissue barrier in implantology, periodentology, endodontics and oral surgery.

BioMet 3i sells a dental product called the NanoTite™ Implant. The screw-shaped device is made of the company's OSSEOTITE® Surface material—which has microscale surface features to encourage bonding. Nanocrystals of calcium phosphate are then bonded to the substrate to help the implant bond even better with bone. This is because calcium is recognized by the body, so it allows for a more natural healing process.

If you need a crown or plan on getting veneers, it's possible you might be getting next-generation teeth—technically called a restoration. Materials used for restoration include acrylic, porcelain, gold, and now, nanomaterials.

3M ESPE was one of the first on the market when they introduced their Filtek™ Supreme Universal Restorative in 2002. The nanocomposite allows for better polishing results (i.e. tooth gloss) and higher strength than traditional materials.

Dialysis

Two treatment options are available to patients with kidney failure: transplantation or dialysis. During hemodialysis, a catheter is inserted into a blood vessel in the arm or leg. The blood is then pumped through an artificial kidney machine containing a filtering system called a dialyzer, which cleans the blood and returns it back to the body. MEMS pressure sensors are used to measure pressure across the filtering membrane. One of the more recent developments comes from Spire Corporation. Their XpressO® and RetrO® hemodialysis catheters are coated with a thin film of nanocrystalline silver to reduce the growth of bacteria. While such catheters are sterile to begin with, once inserted into the body, the ability to further reduce the risk of infection under such circumstances is a continued step forward.

Infusion Pumps/IV Lines

Within the hospital setting, there are three primary means of taking medication: orally (via pills, capsules or liquids), intra-muscular (a "shot") or intravenously (IV). Intravenous medications are provided via IV lines inserted into a vein in the patient (usually the arm or hand). Since the administration of medicine in this manner generally occurs over an extended period of time (from 30 minutes to several days or more), electronic infusion pumps are used for precise and continuous monitoring.

Critically ill patients may be connected to multiple infusion pumps, depending on the number of medicines, nutritional fluids and blood products being administered. The pumps control fluid flowing through the IV tubing. MEMS pressure sensors monitor flow rates and potential blockage.

Needles

The smaller the needle, the less pain experienced when being stuck; but then you run into the possible loss of strength with something so tiny. Micromachining can make needles small, nanotechnology can make them strong. Bioline 1RK91, from Sandvik, is a nanoparticle-based stainless steel that is now being used for ophthalmic, plastic surgery and general suture needles.

Obstetrics/Newborns

MEMS pressure sensors are put to use during delivery in a number of ways; they not only measure intrauterine contraction pressure and frequency, but monitor pressure around the baby's head during delivery.

Right after a baby is born, blood is drawn (typically from the heel) to test bilirubin levels for the detection of jaundice, which is very common in babies. It's often noticeable, since the baby might look yellowish. Bilirubin is produced when red blood cells break down; it's then processed by the liver. Since a baby's liver isn't very mature, it takes longer for this to take place. If necessary, the baby is treated with ultraviolet light to speed the process along.

However, rather than a needle stick, there's actually a non-invasive alternative. The BiliChek® uses a micro-spectrometer to take the same reading without drawing blood. The tip of the device, which looks a lot like an ear thermometer, is briefly placed against the infant's forehead to acquire the data needed.

Ophthalmology

If you don't have an eye exam regularly, you might want to reconsider. Millions of people worldwide have glaucoma, a condition in which the optical nerve is damaged. It is the second leading cause of blindness; the primary reason is that most people are simply unaware that they have the condition. Diabetes is a significant risk factor for this disorder. Only a skilled eye care professional can detect glaucoma early on since there are no changes in vision until the later stages of the disease.

Doctors diagnose glaucoma by detecting increased pressure in the eye (the intraocular pressure or IOP). This is the only, and most significant, symptom. High IOP over a period of time is what damages the optical nerve.

Physical Sciences is using the Multi-DM deformable MEMS mirrors from Boston Micromachines in its adaptive optical spectral domain optical coherence tomography (AO-SDOCT) system. The new product provides better resolution imaging of the human retina to detect and diagnose glaucoma, diabetic retinopathy (spots and blurred vision due to bleeding) and macular degeneration (a loss of your central vision). The mirrors are also used in ophthalmoscopes and LASIK tools for precision steering of the laser beam used to re-shape the cornea.

Orthopedics

Do you know someone who has an artificial joint due to a knee or hip replacement? STRYKER Corporation now sells a number of FDA-approved orthopedic implants with a titanium nanopowder coating to improve longevity. Because the coating enhances tissue growth, the implant is more biocompatible. This is important, since knee and hip joints can be replaced only so many times.

Competitive Technologies sells a bone material based on nanoparticles of calcium phosphate that is used as an easily moldable paste that conforms to host bone (the bone already present in your body that is being fixed). It hardens in ten minutes, can be machined and drilled, and is suitable for both weight and non-weight bearing bones. Having been through a procedure (twice) in which bone is removed from the hip to help fill in a crushed tibia, I can tell you that I'd happily forego the hip surgery in favor of a synthetic bone material instead. However, this material is only being used in conjunction with dental and spinal procedures at this point.

Respirators/Ventilators

MEMS air flow sensors, such as those from Omron, are used to measure gas flow rates and pressure measurement in respirators, oxygen concentrators, ventilators and continuous positive airway pressure (CPAP) masks, which are used by those with severe sleep apnea. The mask is connected to a pump that forces air into the nasal passage to simulate normal breathing. For those who rely on an oxygen tank, pressure sensors monitor oxygen tank levels (just like the tanks for SCUBA divers).

Infection Control

With the outbreak of SARS in 2003, and more recent concerns about the spread of avian flu, companies and government agencies worldwide are taking steps to reduce the risk of infection. This ranges for the obvious (silver nanoparticles) to the not so obvious: infrared sensors.

Thermal imaging cameras from FLIR Systems, based on MEMS microbolometers, are in use in airports around the world for the detection of fever. It's not as strange as it sounds. Fever is a possible indication of infectious disease, such as bird flu. The cameras are also being installed in an increasing number of workplaces for the same reason.

You go to a hospital to get well, but more than 2 million patients in the United States actually get an infection while in a hospital; and more than 70 percent of the bacteria that cause these infections are now resistant to at least one antibiotic[28]. It's no wonder there's been so much focus on the use of silver (either via nanoparticles or ions). Covering surfaces with a coating containing silver makes perfect sense in hospitals.

CMI Enterprises, who manufactures the coated fabrics (think vinyl) used to upholster things like exam tables, wheelchairs, gurneys and chairs, introduced a new line called Dimensions in late 2006. This is the first fabric from the company to leverage its Nanocide™ antimicrobial. Able to kill 99.9 percent of resistant staph bacteria that comes in contact with it, the fabrics do indeed use silver nanoparticles.

Trevira sells a line of fabrics called Trevira Bioactive, which is being used for things like drapes, surgical gowns, scrubs and other textiles within the hospital setting. Their approach relies on the use of silver ions though, not nanoparticles.

Perhaps the most important angle to infection control is patients with large wounds (those bigger than you can put a bandage on). In this case, sterile dressings are critical, because the risk of infection is so high. Silver was used long before the introduction of antibiotics, and is regaining in popularity.

One of the first to address this from a nanotech perspective was NUCRYST. The Acticoat™ Antimicrobial Barrier Dressings rely on the company's nanocrystalline technology (SILCRYST™), which is comprised of silver crystals between 1 and 100 nanometers in size. However, the dressings release silver ions over a period of time, which is another example of how the distinction between nano-particles and silver ions can blur.

Johnson & Johnson takes a slightly different approach with their SILVERCEL dressings, which rely on the use of silver-coated fibers, like those from Noble Fiber Technologies. I point this product out because it entered the market at about the same time as the CURAD® Silver bandages, so there was considerable discussion about the use of ions and nanoparticles at that time; in this case, neither was correct.

Nanofibers are also finding their way into dressings. The Nanospider™ technology from Nanopeutics is used in a product called m.doc™ (Micro Dispersed Oxidized Cellulose), which helps to stop bleeding and promote healing.

Pharmaceuticals

There's considerable nanotechnology-oriented research taking place as it pertains to pharmaceuticals. It's believed that the formation of drugs at the nanoscale will make them more effective with fewer side effects. While many products are currently in clinical trials, one has FDA approval: ABRAXANE® (from Abraxis BioScience), which is used for the treatment of advanced breast cancer. However, the particles of this drug are *nanoscale*, or about 130 nanometers. While this is an exciting area to watch, MEMS and nanotechnology are already making a difference in the delivery of medicine into the body, as well as the production of pharmaceuticals themselves.

Drug Delivery

The pharmaceuticals you take to make you well can be administered in all sorts of innovative ways:

- Inhale it—like asthma medicine
- Drop it into your eyes
- Swallow it—in pill, capsule, tablet or liquid form
- Wear it like a patch—so it's absorbed through the skin
- Inject it—as a "shot"

How are MEMS playing a role? A transdermal drug delivery system from ALZA called Macroflux® is based on a thin titanium screen with tiny microprojections (micromachined needles). The MEMS needles that are part of this patch help medicine better penetrate the skin. Because they're so small, you won't feel them.

If you've had a surgical procedure, in some instances you may be sent home with a catheter that continuously administers a local anesthetic for non-narcotic pain relief. These are only typically in place for just a few days. However, as with any such device, there's always the risk of infection at the insertion site.

The ON-Q SilverSoaker™ anesthesia delivery catheter from I-Flow Corporation has a coating containing silver nanoparticles to reduce the risk of infection. The FDA approved it in late 2005.

Drug Production

I never really gave much thought to how pharmaceuticals are produced. But as it turns out, micro-spectrometers are being put to use as a quality control tool. Thermo Electron's Antaris™ Target Blend Analyzer controls blend uniformity. If you think about it, that's pretty important. Medicine is a combination of active ingredients (the actual drug) and inactive ingredients (which add bulk, color, flavoring, preservation, etc). Maintaining the right balance between the two is important so that you don't end up with one pill that's all active ingredients and another that is all inactive ingredients.

It's along the lines of making chocolate chip cookies. You want the chips distributed as evenly as possible throughout the cookie dough, so that each cookie has the right balance of dough and chips. Too few chips in one cookie, or too many in another, wouldn't meet the set quality control standards of manufacturers.

The use of a tool to make sure that products are mixed consistently throughout may not be important to cookie-making at home, but it's certainly important for industrial manufacturing.

As for the production of nanoemulsions (like the ones used in cosmetics), I think many will be surprised to learn that MEMS devices are actually behind the emulsification process. A company by the name of Microfluidics sells a product called the Multiple Stream Mixer Reactor, which relies on their Microfluidizer® technology. This allows companies to manufacture emulsions, dispersions, liposomes and other similar products.

The approach is basically the same as lab-on-a-chip, where microchannels and chambers are put to use. In this case, highly pressurized fluids flow through two different microchannels into a single chamber where they collide and mix together. The use of high pressure (up to 40,000 pounds per square inch) and velocity (or speed) helps to ensure this. The material then exits through a single microchannel. Flow sensors monitor the rate of flow through the channels.

Hitachi Plant Technologies introduced a similar system in early 2007. If you think this is a huge room-size piece of equipment, think again. Go get your wallet. To put this system into perspective, the device they use is about the size of a credit card. One of their target applications is the production of oil-water emulsions, something that's now easier due to the use of nanoscale materials.

Yum, it's been light-years since you programmed synthetic brownies.

—*George Jetson (The Jetsons, 1962)*

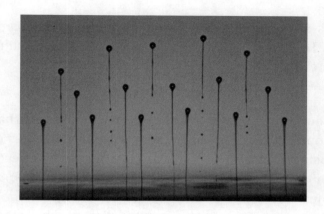

12 • WHERE ELSE ARE NANO/MEMS FOUND?

Have you ever seen the now-classic movie "Willy Wonka and the Chocolate Factory?" Watch it again when you have the chance; it provides an insightful look into how products are made. Industrial manufacturing may not seem like a very interesting topic, but the movie does put it into a whole new perspective. My point is that MEMS and nanotechnology are at work in places that the general public will likely never see; yet, they still have a direct effect on your daily life.

Look around you. Do you fly in an airplane once in a while? Buy frozen vegetables or prepared dinners? Drink beer? Play poker? Go to movies? Have you ever wondered how oil is found? How paper is made? How the water treatment plant in your city makes water drinkable? Industrial processing is a central part of our lives, whether we realize it or not. And both MEMS and nanomaterials are making those processes smarter, faster and more efficient. Let's take a look at some applications that I think you'll find interesting.

Aerospace

Did you know that some airline seats now have airbags—just like the ones in cars? In early 2007, Singapore Airlines outfitted every business and first class seat on a number of new aircraft with AmSafe's Aviation Inflatable Restraint (AAIR®) system. They're just the latest airline to take advantage of the system, which the company introduced in 2001. Part of the seatbelt itself, the protection system is already included in light aircraft built by Cessna and CIRRUS Design, as well as some flights operated by Virgin Atlantic Airways and nearly two dozen other commercial airlines. They're generally part of the seatbelts worn by the crew, but are slowly finding their way into passenger seats.

Food

The massive, national recall of Peter Pan Peanut Butter (due to Salmonella) and numerous brands of pet food (due to the industrial ingredient melamine) in early 2007 in the United States highlights the need for better quality control tools within the food industry. But companies such as Biacore (now part of GE Healthcare), already offer such products. Their microfluidic chip technology is currently used to ensure consistent vitamin content in fortified foods, testing for antibiotics in honey and screening for veterinary drug residue in livestock and poultry.

While the use of MEMS in food safety is clearly a good thing, the impending creation of "nanofood" is generating a lot of controversy. It's been widely reported for years that food giants Altria, Heinz, Kraft, Nestle and Unilever are conducting considerable research in this area. But the term is more than a little misleading, because most people probably assume that means nanoparticle-based ice cream or soda. At this point, what we're really looking at are things along the line of nanotech-based films and bottles used to package food.

Controversy is nothing new to food. In 2002, concerns arose about the use of irradiation, a type of sterilization technique used to kill bacteria in food, as well as extend shelf life; but the FDA approved it for use back in 1972. The issue came about when the FDA considered expanding the use of irradiation. This was due, in part, to a series of massive food recalls in the late 1990s, affecting millions of pounds of ground beef, hot dogs and deli meat. That's what brought the topic into the public eye, resulting in some big-time opposition. Just a year later, the controversy was forgotten.

We've been playing with our food, seeking new ways to make it safer and taste better, for as long as we've been eating. Today, more than 3,000 substances (things to improve taste, texture, appearance and preservation) are approved for the direct addition to food[29]. But, the list includes things like herbs and spices, as well as additives used for centuries, such as salt and vinegar; how else do you make pickles?

The list also includes vitamins and minerals; another area of some controversy. Most salt today is iodized, due to the addition of iodine, which began in the 1920s. In the 1930s, vitamin D was added to milk. Since the 1940s, white flour and bread have been enriched with iron, thiamin (B_1), riboflavin (B_2) and niacin (B_3). In the 1980s, calcium was added to all sorts of products, such as orange juice. Why? Modern food processing strips the nutrients from the original ingredients; so they're added in after-the-fact.

It is true that nanoscale food ingredients are being developed; some are already available and in use. But like cosmetics, there's a gray area here between nanotechnology, nanoscale and even basic chemistry. After reading Chapter 8, we now know that lipids are nanoscale. In the food industry, lipids are another word for fat, which as we all know, is a very common ingredient (think of all of the cooking oils you can buy). But, did you know that when we make some foods, nanostructures naturally form? You and I have no control over that, and we wouldn't even know without the use of the special equipment that now tells us this is so; just like the ancient metalworkers forging Damascus steel.

Starch, a carbohydrate made from things like corn, potatoes or rice, is also a common food thickening agent. Although the Egyptians used starch as glue, it's believed that the ancient Greeks and Romans were the first to use it in the preparation of food[30]. If you make sauces or gravies at home, by thickening them with flour, the concept is the same. Cornstarch (starch made from corn) differs in that it thickens faster than flour, has no taste and results in a much smoother consistency. Plus, it can be used to thicken both cold and hot foods. When making jams, jellies, curds, custards, sauces and similar products, the cooking and cooling process results in the melting and re-crystallization of carbohydrates at the nanoscale[31].

As far as ingredients go (nano or otherwise), the general point is to improve product taste and texture, as well as nutritional content. AQUANOVA provides a good representative example of the application of nanotechnology to food. The company's product, NovaSOL®, is a nanosome about 30 nanometers in diameter. You already know that a nanosome is a liposome, or a naturally-occurring lipid. Because it's hollow, it can be filled with ingredients. In this case, those ingredients include things like vitamin A, beta-carotene, vitamin C, citric acid, ascorbic acid, vitamin E, Omega-3 and sorbic acid. These are all ingredients already found in most prepared foods for decades; just read the nutrition label.

Why go nanoscale? As with cosmetics, it allows manufacturers to combine ingredients that weren't possible before (think of the nanoemulsions), as well as adding ingredients to end-use products that you otherwise couldn't. One example is a white bread that contains nanoencapsulated Omega-3. Why? Because fish oil is good for you; in this case, it increases the bread's nutritional factor without the fishy taste commonly associated with Omega-3. I suspect a new era of food enrichment is going to be the controversy here; not the use of nanotechnology per se.

Beyond ingredients, there's a new piece of equipment for use in cooking food. Called the OilFresh™ 1000, it's a thin ceramic plate that goes into the deep fat fryers in restaurants. Commercial fryers are large, rectangular, metal bins that look a little bit like a kichen sink, which holds the hot oil used to cook. Baskets containing food are the lowered into the bins and cooked.

In busy kitchens, especially those in fast food restaurants, there's a lot of frying going on. Over the course of several days of use, the oil starts to break down. As a result, oil molecules start clumping together; it's not going bad, the food simply takes longer to cook. This is why french fries can be a light golden brown one day, and a slightly darker brown on another day.

Made of nanoceramics, it you looked at the plate really closely, it might remind you of a sponge. What it does is slow the break-down of the oil; so restaurants can fry food faster, at a slightly lower temperature. The bottom line is that restaurants use less oil, which of course, saves them money. But, since foods fry faster, that means they won't absorb as much oil, making them slightly healthier (if it's possible to say that about fried food).

Food Packaging

Nanocomposites are finding some of their most useful applications in food packaging. Next time you're at the grocery store (in the U.S., anyway), take a close look at how extensively plastic is used; from the films that enclose meat and pre-packaged foods, to the bottles lining the shelves. What role do nanocomposites play? They improve the barrier of plastic films and bottles; that means that air can't penetrate, so food stays fresher, longer. They're already being used to create next-generation containers for deli meats and films for potato chip bags (to keep them crisp).

One of the more interesting applications of nanocomposites I mentioned in Chapter 3 is plastic beer bottles. One reason that beer is sold in glass bottles is because air molecules can't diffuse, or move in and out of glass. That means beer stays carbonated. You would think the same problem holds true for soda (which is sold in large, plastic bottles), but apparently the issue is of greater concern with beer. One reason why the brewing industry is so interested in the use of plastic bottles (which they've looked into for years) is that they cost much less than glass.

Beer bottles made of nanocomposites made their debut in 2006, courtesy of Coors and AMCOL. Hite Brewery and Honeywell also worked together to create a plastic beer bottle. In some instances, the entire bottle is made of a nanocomposite, in other instances, the nanocomposite is a barrier material; an internal coating that is used in conjunction with conventional plastics.

Next-generation plastic wrap, and the plastic film on packaged food, is coming courtesy of SKC. Their Fancylite color film doesn't use dyes or pigments; instead it's made up of hundreds of individual layers, each just a few nanometers thick. The color of each layer depends on how thick it is; the final color of the plastic film depends on how many layers there are. Rather than being a solid color, the film will have an iridescent or rainbow-like effect, depending on the light and viewing angle.

Another packaging material where nanotechnology is already in play is cardboard. Again, look closely at the extensive use of boxes used to package everything from cereal to ice cream. Cardboard is made up of layers of paper glued to each other; the glossy, finished layer (with all of the graphics) is laminated, or glued on top.

A new adhesive made from nanoparticles of starch is keeping labels and other graphics stuck to fast food containers. As you just read, starch is widely used as an ingredient in all sorts of food. Developed by Ecosynthetix, the approach is also environmentally friendly; since there's more surface area to the particles, the adhesive requires less water, so it dries faster. Plus, it's biodegradable, whereas the glues typically used right now aren't since they're petroleum-based.

Food Production

Food processing is highly water-intensive. Processing plants use water to rinse raw materials such as vegetables (often multiple times during different steps), to prepare food (such as during slicing), to carry raw materials down the line to the next step, as a principal ingredient and in sanitizing, not only of the food itself, but the equipment used throughout the entire process. One large food processing plant can easily use more than 1 million gallons of water per day, resulting in very large waste streams. The water was drinkable to start with, but it certainly isn't after all is said and done. What to do?

Food processing plants are looking to their waste streams as a way to generate electricity. NanoLogix is making this happen with their hydrogen bioreactor, which creates hydrogen from the waste stream, which is then converted into electricity for use by the processing facility. Such a system is in use at a Welch Foods plant.

How does it work? In a word—bacteria. That's more than a little ironic, considering how many companies are now using all forms of silver to kill the microscopic critters. But, bacteria are actually used in waste streams to help make water treatment easier. In the case of the NanoLogix system, the basic concept is this: bacteria eat organic matter found in the waste stream, and in this case, release carbon dioxide and hydrogen. The hydrogen is then harnessed and converted to electricity.

Another new use of nanotechnology in conjunction with food processing is nano-bubbles. That's right, nano-bubbles. The RVK-N1 from Royal Electric combines nano-bubbles of ozone with micro-bubbles of an ozone/oxygen mix. It's used to clean seafood.

Marubeni Corporation sells a similar device for use in waste-water treatment. Given all of the water used within food processing facilities, manufacturers have a lot of wastewater to manage. Increasing the amount of air in wastewater makes it easier to culture the bacteria needed to eat the organic material.

Entertainment

Counterfeiting is a huge problem. The one item that most people think of in this respect is probably money. But the issue ranges from luxury goods, such as design purses and watches, to things you might not consider, like pharmaceuticals. Generally, the higher the value of something, the more likely it's going to be knocked-off, or counterfeited. In some instances, the difference between a real item and a fake item are very difficult to identify, and in other instances, it's really obvious.

What does this have to do with entertainment? A new anti-counterfeiting technology called DataTraceDNA is being applied to high value poker chips. Despite the name, and the fact that it's been referred to as a molecular barcode, it has nothing to do with the human body. Rather, the technology is added to the plastic used to manufacture the chips. Because product identification is part of the molecular structure of the plastic itself, it's extremely difficult for counterfeiters to figure out and replicate. So, next time you're at a poker table in Las Vegas, you might have a really ingenious application of nanotechnology sitting right in front of you.

If movies are your thing, you can enjoy the use of Texas Instruments' DLP® at your local theater. More than 3,200 theaters in 30 countries (and growing fast) now show movies on projectors that use the chips (resulting in better picture quality and more vivid colors). The chances are good that one is in your neighborhood. Plus, more companies are using the technology during movie post-production (i.e. editing); so watching a digitally-created movie on a digital projector means that movies will always look pristine. The days of watching movies with faded color, scratches on the film and occasional jitter as the film moves through the projector, are over.

Speaking of movies, do you ever wonder how today's computer generated characters in movies and video games move so realistically? Actors wear special suits embedded with sensors to track their movements. The GypsyGyro line of motion capture suits from Animazoo use the InertiaCube™ (a combination of a MEMS gyro sensor and accelerometers) from InterSense to precisely track both linear and rotational movement of the actor's body. This makes motion capture really precise, which is why computer generated characters move much more realistically than they did even a few years ago.

Oil & Gas Production

There's a lot of talk about the eventual use of nanotechnology for next-generation solar technology. But both MEMS and nano-materials are playing very important roles today in all aspects of oil & gas exploration and production.

MEMS are key components in geophysical services—the exploration for oil. Geophones, a type of MEMS sensor developed by Sercel, help to find oil deposits by using sound to create a map of underground structures by detecting ground motion. The earth is made up of different layers, each of which sends back a slightly different signal. In this case, geologists can see what layer is rock, what might be water, and where oil is located, depending on the data the sensors send back.

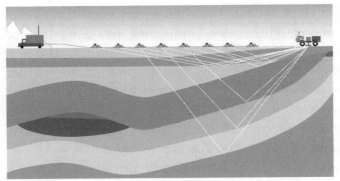

Creating a map of the earth's layers. Illustration courtesy of Sercel.

Accelerometers are used in advanced seismic data systems (i.e. seismic survey planning, design, data acquisition), which are critical to managing the risk of oil exploration—you don't necessarily want to place oil wells in an area prone to a lot of movement of the earth, which would damage the structures. Both accelerometers and pressure sensors are also important components in oil drilling, as well as production processes.

Nanotechnology is also making a strong move in the oil and gas sector—aerogels are insulating pipelines, nano-based catalysts improve processing, nanofibers offer more selective filtering, and of course, nanocomposites offer stronger, lighter materials for drilling equipment and pipelines.

Speaking of pipelines, the news in late 2006 about the shut down and subsequent replacement of 16 miles of petroleum giant BP plc's pipeline in Prudhoe Bay, Alaska (due to the effects of corrosion), serves to highlight the role MEMS and nanotech could have played in possibly preventing the problem in the first place.

Take into consideration the environment these pipelines are operating in—rain, snow, ice, freezing and thawing—all of which can wreak havoc on pipe insulation, making it vulnerable to cracking. As a result, water is able to penetrate and start the corrosion process. Next-generation insulation materials, based on aerogels, are not only available, but specifically targeting oil pipelines.

If insulation isn't enough, how about backing it up with a coating product that specifically protects against corrosion? Such a product does indeed exist, although Industrial Nanotech was initially targeting low temperature pipes in industrial and manufacturing plants. In fact, Brazilian oil company Petrobas is now using the coating as part of its maintenance program.

Of course, the whole issue with BP came about due to the fact that they had not regularly used maintenance pigs (plastic cylinders that scrape away the sludge build-up that occurs) to clean out the pipelines, thus allowing for internal corrosion.

"Smart pigs" are also typically used, which have the ability to detect corrosion using magnetic and/or ultrasonic sensing, as they move through the pipeline. MEMS pressure and flow sensors, and even a viscometer (such as the one from Convergence Ethanol) can detect minute changes in oil flow, thus pinpointing a sludge build-up issue far more quickly.

Beyond protecting oil pipelines, nanomaterials are also protecting consumers at the gas station. In some countries, fuel such as gas and kerosone is sometimes improperly diluted with cheaper ingredients, resulting in inferior fuel sold at a premium price. But counterfeit fuel can be damaging to cars and other equipment.

Authentix has a solution. They've developed a unique "nano-marker" which, when blended into fuel with other fuel addititives, results in a unique chemical signature that is trackable. Their product doesn't alter the quality or performance of the gas; rather, it simply allows inspectors to check the fuel's authenticity right at the retail pump. This assures that customers are getting what they're paying for.

Paper

The use of nanoparticles in the paper-making process actually got its start in the late 1980s for the production of what's called fine paper; this is generally the smooth, white paper used by consumers, compared to the rougher textured paper used for newspapers, and the even rougher paper layers of cardboard. Today, more than 350 machines in 25 countries produce paper based on silica nanoparticles; as a result, it's a high probability that nearly all fine papers today now contain nanoparticles.

I know what you're thinking: how on earth can nanoparticles make a difference here? Paper is paper, right? Not to the people who make it, or the printers who use it. The average consumer may not realize this, but the use of nanoparticles results in paper of a higher quality that's easier to print on, with better results. In addition, these papers are not only lighter, but they have much greater stiffness. In the past, paper stiffness was a direct result of how thick it was. Lightweight paper had little stiffness in comparison —until now.

Paper is made from a mixture of wood fibers (which are expensive), along with various chemicals and fillers. The addition of silica nanoparticles improves, among other things, paper quality and strength. The end result is a paper surface that's smooth and even. Plus, the use of nanoparticles significantly reduces the amount of raw materials needed, which ultimately saves trees.

Akzo Nobel is a leader in this area with its Compozil® family of products, which it launched in 1980.

In early 2007, Mondi Business Paper began selling a new line of paper called neox. What makes this paper special? It uses the NanoTope paper coating from TopChim. The result is a nano-structured surface, which results in a cross between the gloss and smooth feel of coated paper, with the whiteness and stiffness of uncoated paper. The result is a more versatile paper—especially for color laser printing.

Space Exploration

The original Mars rover—Sojourner—used a MEMS gyro sensor to help it navigate, and aerogels insulated the fragile electronics from the sub-zero temperature on the red planet. As NASA prepared to launch their next-generation rovers they developed a test rover called FIDO (Field Integrated Design Operations) to test theories about the martian environment, so the new rovers could be as prepared as possible; it also used a MEMS gyro sensor.

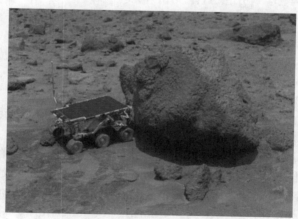

Photo courtesy of NASA/JPL-Caltech

The two newest rovers, Spirit and Opportunity, both benefit from the protection of aerogel-based insulation. This may partially explain why they've lasted so long, despite the extremely cold temperature on the planet Mars.

MEMS hydrogen sensors from Makel Engineering were demonstrated on Space Shuttle Discovery in 1997, as the well as a number of discontinued projects, including the X33 Space Plane, the X43 Hypersonic Jet and the Helios Fly Wing. In all cases, the sensor's job was to detect potential hydrogen leaks. They're currently in place in the International Space Station to monitor hydrogen levels in the oxygen regeneration system.

In late 2006, the U.S. Air Force Research Laboratory launched their TacSat-2 satellite. On board was an instrument called the Inertial Stellar Compass (ISC), which is part of the Space Technology 6 Project. ISC is a miniature star-tracking camera and MEMS gyro suite which takes pictures of the stars and then compares them to onboard maps of the solar system. The device is meant for use in future spacecraft to determine its orientation, or where it is—it's a bit like GPS for space.

In early 2007, the Air Force Academy launched the Falconsat-3 microsatellite on a six-month mission to better understand plasma bubbles (the depletion of plasma in the ionosphere). This is important because such incidents can disrupt satellite communications. On board is a Flat Plasma Spectrometer (FlaPS), built by researchers at Johns Hopkins University. The micro-spectrometer will help collect and analyze the necessary data.

When NASA's three Space Technology 5 (ST5) satellites launched (also in early 2007), one of them was outfitted with a unique MEMS device meant to control its temperature. The Variable Emittance (Vari-E) Coating for Thermal Control looks like a microscopic version of the wood shutters you might have on your windows except, in this case, they're silicon. Just like in your home, the shutters open and close to maintain a constant temperature (here, they do so automatically). So, when facing the sun, the shutters close to reflect the heat; to absorb more heat, the shutters open to let the light (and heat) in.

A lab-on-a-chip device from Lionix BV is part of the European Space Agency's upcoming ExoMars Mission, where it will be used to analyze Martian soil. Micro-spectrometers from Polychromix are part of NASA's planned Lunar Crater Observation and Sensing Satellite (LCROSS), in which they will identify the presence of water ice at the moon's South Pole.

One of the largest MEMS deformable mirrors ever built is being integrated into the UCO/Lick Observatory, located at the University of California Santa Cruz. From Boston Micromachines, it will help in the study of extra-solar planets as part of the Gemini Planet Imager. The company's deformable mirrors are also part of NASA's Terrestial Planet Finder Mission and the Extrasolar Planet Imaging Coronograph Discovery mission.

Water

With all of the talk about food-borne illness, would it help to know that both MEMS and nanotechnology are being used to keep our water supplies safe? I bet you don't even consider the potential risks there. The BioSentry™ system from JMAR Technologies uses lasers to monitor, detect and classify whether microorganisms (such cryptosporidium, giardia, E. coli, salmonella, shigella, and legionella) are present in water. It's being used in places where it makes a lot of sense: during the production of products such as purified water, carbonated drinks, juices and other beverages, and even on cruise ships.

Lab-on-a-chip is also quickly finding its way into municipal water plants. The WaterPOINT™ handheld system from Sensicore allows workers to check water for things like chlorine, pH, conductivity and alkalinity (plus ten other water parameters), and provides results back in just four minutes. Being able to conduct these tests much more quickly makes the water treatment process far more efficient.

What's Next?

The purpose of this book is to discuss real products on the market today—there are plenty of news stories about the "imagine this" and "what ifs" of nanotechnology. But there's so much in the development pipeline that I thought it would be fun to provide a glimpse of the kinds of things we can expect to see on the market in the not-too-distant future.

- DataTraceDNA is developing a multi-color barcode (based on its molecular barcode technology) for use in conjunction with DVDs, video games and other media, to prevent the sale of counterfeit products.

- GE is developing a superhydrophobic plastic. Just think—a plastic bottle where you can get the last bit of ketchup out just as easily as the first.

- Introgen Therapeutics is working with Colgate-Palmolive to develop a line of nano-formulated oral rinses and other similar products for the prevention and/or treatment of pre-cancerous conditions of the mouth.

- Mediscience is developing the Biopsy Pill for the detection of pre-cancerous and cancerous tissue in the digestive tract.

- MicroCHIPS is developing a fully implantable MEMS chip for the long-term, time-release delivery of drugs.

- Novo Nordisk is in Phase 3 clinical trials with an inhaled insulin product that leverages the AERx Strip™ technology from Aradigm Corporation. The disposable strip is an array of laser-micromachined nozzles, each of which is just 1 micron in diameter.

- Pharmos Corporation completed Phase 1 studies of its nanoemulsion of diclofenac, a widely used, non-steroidal, anti-inflammatory drug (NSAID). The company plans to use it as a topical cream for the treatment of pain associated with osteoarthritis.

- pSivida is in Phase II clinical trials of BrachySil™, an implantable drug delivery system for the treatment of inoperable primary liver cancer. It relies on a unique nanostructure that is biocompatible and biodegradable.

- SAVR Communications is developing a package-level device which will monitor the temperature, fluid level, light, radiation and humidity conditions of high value goods as they're shipped via DHL. Accelerometers will let you know if it's been dropped.

- Second Sight® Medical Products is in clinical studies with their Argus™ II retinal Prosthesis System. The implantable MEMS array helps some people with substantial vision loss to see again.

- Star Pharma's VivaGel™, a dendrimer-based gel to protect women against sexually-transmitted disease, is currently in clinical trials.

- US Global Nanotech is developing a nanofiber-based cigarette filter called the NanoFilterCX™.

GLOSSARY

Accelerometer—a sensor that measures linear motion

Aerogel—a material made of nanoscale pockets of air

Atom—the basic building block of life, an atom is about one-third of a nanometer in diameter

Atomic Force Microscope (AFM)—a tool that allows for the imaging of nano- and micro-scale objects in detail

Buckyball (see *fullerene*)

Cantilever—a MEMS structure that looks like a diving board

Carbon Nanotube—a cylindrical, tube-like arrangement of carbon atoms, about 1 nanometer in diameter, that looks like a roll of chicken wire

Dendrimer—a synthetic, three-dimensional molecule, just a few nanometers in diameter, that looks like a snowflake

Fullerene—a molecular cluster of pure carbon that looks like a soccer ball and is also called a buckyball

Gyro—a MEMS sensor that measures rotational motion

Hydrophilic—attracts water

Hydrophobic—repels water

IMU (Inertial measurement unit)—the combination of an accelerometer and gyro sensor to measure both linear and rotational movement

Inertial sensor—a MEMS sensor that measures motion

Infrared sensor—a MEMS device that measures heat

Ion—a charged atom or molecule

Lab-on-a-chip—a MEMS device that moves fluid through an array of tiny channels

Liposome—a naturally-occurring lipid (fat) used to carry other liquids, much like a water balloon, but with the consistency of a soap bubble

Lotus effect—the ability to self-clean (see *self-cleaning effect*)

Magnetic compass—the use of an accelerometer and magnetic sensor to monitor motion and direction

MEMS—three-dimensional objects that perform a mechanical function, whose dimensions are between 1 to 100 micrometers

Microbolometer—a MEMS device that measures infrared radiation

Microfabricated (see *micromachined*)

Microfluidics—the movement of fluid through structures with dimensions less than 100 micrometers

Micromachined—a general term for the fabrication of MEMS

Microspectrometer—a MEMS device that measures light

Molecule—the combination of two or more atoms; generally smaller than one nanometer in diameter

Nanoclay—a particle of nanoscale clay

Nanocomposite—a material (typically plastic) with nano-particles mixed in to make it lighter and stronger

Nanofiber—fibers at the nanoscale; they're spun like cotton candy

Nanomaterial—a material (in liquid, powder or solid form) whose particles are nanoscale

Nanoparticle—a particle of material at the nanoscale

Nanoscale—a form of measurement pertaining to objects with dimensions between 1 and 999 nanometers

Nanoscience—the study of nanoscale objects

Nanosilver—a nanoscale particle of silver

Nanotechnology—a material or structure purposefully manu-factured with dimensions between 1 and 100 nanometers to leverage the unique properties it has at the size

OLED (Organic light emitting diode)—a type of color display made up of several layers of different materials, a little bit like a sandwich

Optical MEMS—a MEMS device that moves light

POC (Point-of-care Diagnostics)—a chip used to test blood

Printhead—a chip containing an array of nozzles (or holes) through which ink moves during ink jet printing

Quantum Dot—a one-nanometer piece of a silicon wafer

RF MEMS—a class of MEMS devices used to make electronics work better

Self-cleaning effect—the ability of water droplets to roll off a surface, taking dust and other particles with them, thus leaving the surface clean

Shear thickening fluid—a fluid comprised of nanoparticles that becomes rigid (hard) upon impact

Strain gauge—a MEMS device that senses weight

Sub-micron—an object or structure with dimensions between 100 and 900 nanometers (0.1 micrometers to 0.9 micrometers)

Thermopile—a MEMS device that measures heat

Vesicle—a liposome (see *liposome*)

REFERENCES

1—ASTM International, "E 2456, Terminology for Nanotechnology," December 2006.

2—C. S. Smith, "Piezoresistance Effect in Germanium and Silicon," *Phys. Rev.*, vol. 94, no. 1 (1954): 42-49.

3—R. Feynman, "There's Plenty of Room at the Bottom," American Physical Society Annual Meeting, California Institute of Technology, 1959.

4—N. Taniguchi, "On the basic concept of nano-technology," Japan Society of Precision Engineering, Tokyo, 1974.

5—Texas Instruments, "A History of Innovation," www.dlp.com.

6—M. McCulloch et al, "Diagnostic Accuracy of Canine Scent Detection in Early- and Late-Stage Lung and Breast Cancers," *Integrative Cancer Therapies*, 5(1) (2006): 30-9.

7—British Broadcasting Corporation, "On This Day | 30 | 1986: Coal mine canaries made redundant," December 30, 1986.

8—S. Robinson, "The Chicken Defense," *Time Magazine*, February 21, 2003.

9—J. Goreva et al, "Fibrous nanoinclusions in massive rose quartz: The origin of rose coloration," *American Mineralogist* 86 (2001): 466-472.

10—M. José-Yacamàn et al, "Maya Blue Paint: An Ancient Nano-structured Material," *Science*, Vol. 273, No. 5272 (12 July 1996): 223-225.

11—M. Reibold et al, "Carbon nanotubes in an ancient Damascus saber," *Nature*, 444 (2006): 286.

12—Robert J. Blazej, Palani Kumaresan and Richard A. Mathies, "Microfabricated bioprocessor for integrated nanoliter-scale Sanger DNA sequencing", *PNAS* 103 (2006): 7240-7245.

13—US Department of State and the Department of Health and Human Services National Institute on Aging, National Institutes of Health, "Why Population Aging Matters: A Global Perspective," March 2007.

14—National Center for Health Statistics, Centers for Disease Control and Prevention, US Department of Health and Human Services, "NHANES data on the Prevalence of Overweight and Obesity Among Adults-United States, 2003-2004."

15—National Center for Health Statistics, Centers for Disease Control and Prevention, US Department of Health and Human Services, "Prevalence of Overweight Among Children and Adolescents: United States, 2003-2004."

16—World Health Organization, http://www.who.int, April 2007.

17, 19, 23—National Center for Health Statistics, Centers for Disease Control and Prevention, US Department of Health and Human Services, "Summary Health Statistics for U.S. Adults: National Health Interview Survey, 2005."

18, 21—National Center for Health Statistics, Centers for Disease Control and Prevention, US Department of Health and Human Services, "Health, United States, 2006."

20—National Center for Health Statistics, Centers for Disease Control and Prevention, US Department of Health and Human Services, "Summary Health Statistics for U.S. Children: National Health Interview Survey, 2005."

22—Bethany Halford, "Nanotech Makes Your Brown Eyes Blue," *Chemical & Engineering News*, Volume 83, Number 41 (October 10, 2005): 42-43.

24—National Institute on Deafness and Other Communication Disorders, National Institutes of Health, "Statistics about Hearing Disorders, Ear Infections, and Deafness," April 2007.

25—National Diabetes Information Clearinghouse, National Institute of Diabetes and Digestive and Kidney Disease, National Institutes of Health, "Total Prevalence of Diabetes in the United States, All Ages, 2005."

26—National Center for Health Statistics, Centers for Disease Control and Prevention, US Department of Health and Human Services, "National Hospital Ambulatory Medical Care Survey: 2004 Emergency Department Summary," June 2006.

27—A. Bobbio, "Maya, the first authentic alloplastic, endosseous dental implant. A refinement of a priority" *Rev Assoc Paul Cir Dent*, Jan-Feb 27(1) (1973): 27-36.

28—Department of Health and Human Services, Centers for Disease Control and Prevention, "Antimicrobial Resistance in Healthcare Settings," April 2007.

29—Center for Food Safety and Applied Nutrition, US Food and Drug Administration, "Everything Added to Food in the United States (EAFUS)," April 2007.

30—William R. Mason, "100 Years of Food Starch Technology," National Starch and Chemical Company.

31—VJ Morris, "Probing molecular interactions in foods," *Trends in Food Science & Technology* 15 (2004): 291-297.

32—P. Coleman Saunders, Victoria Interrante and Sean C. Garrick, "Pointillist and Glyph-Based Visualization of Nanoparticles in Formation," *Joint Eurographics/IEEE-VGTC Symposium on Visualization* (2005): 169-176.

33—Robert J. Blazej, Palani Kumaresan and Richard A. Mathies, "Microfabricated bioprocessor for integrated nanoliter-scale Sanger DNA sequencing," *PNAS* 103 (2006): 7240-7245.

34—N.S. Cameron, M.K. Corbierre and A. Eisenberg, "Asymmetric amphiphilic block copolymers in solution: A morphological wonderland," *Can. J. Chem.* 77 (1999): 1311-1326.

ADDITIONAL PHOTO CREDITS

Page 23—Photo of "MEMS Gear" courtesy of Sandia National Laboratories, SUMMiT™ Technologies, www.mems.sandia.gov.

Page 43—Photo of "Gold Nanoparticles" reproduced by kind permission of the Eurographics Association; © 2005 Eurographics Assocation. P. Coleman Saunders, Victoria Interrante and Sean C. Garrick, "Pointillist and Glyph-Based Visualization of Nanoparticles in Formation," *Joint Eurographics/IEEE-VGTC Symposium on Visualization* (2005): 169-176.

Page 67—Photo of "Nanohand and its Captured Ball" taken by Dr. Jack Luo and Dr. Yong Qing Fu, Department of Engineering at the University of Cambridge. The image is part of the Epson Photography Competition at the Department of Engineering at the University of Cambridge (www.eng.cam.ac.uk). The competition is sponsored by Epson (www.epson.co.uk).

Page 81—Photo of "Micro-car" courtesy of DENSO Corporation.

Page 103—Photo of "Nanowire Forest" courtesy of Oak Ridge National Laboratory (Dr. Zhenwei Pan).

Page 127—Photo of "Nanoguitar" courtesy of Harold Craighead, Cornell University.

Page 145—Photo of "Pregnant Vesicles" courtesy of NRC Press. N.S. Cameron, M.K. Corbierre and A. Eisenberg, "Asymmetric amphiphilic block copolymers in solution: A morphological wonderland," *Can. J. Chem.* 77 (1999): 1311-1326.

Page 171—Photo of "Butterfly Pendant" courtesy of Sensory Design and Technology Ltd.

Page 189—Computer generated image of a buckyball courtesy of Lawrence Berkeley National Laboratory.

Page 215—Photo of "Self-Assembled Silver Nanowires" courtesy of Ward Lopes and Heinrich Jaeger, University of Chicago.

Page 245—Photo of "Tails from the nozzle bank" taken by Dr. Steve Hoath, Department of Engineering at the University of Cambridge. The image is part of the Epson Photography Competition at the Department of Engineering at the University of Cambridge (www.eng.cam.ac.uk). The competition is sponsored by Epson (www.epson.co.uk).

INDEX

3M, 123, 171
3M ESPE, 235

A

A123Systems, 88, 89, 113
Abraxis BioScience, 241
accelerometers, 14, 16, 26, 28,
    29, 30, 41, 83, 85–87, 98, 99,
    104, 107, 118, 129, 131–133,
    135–138, 140, 141, 143, 190,
    191, 194, 196, 197, 198, 202,
    203, 205, 207, 208, 221–223,
    226, 253, 254, 261, 264
AccuFLEX, 202
ACRALIGHT International
    Skylights, 123
active suspension, 84
adhesives, 59
adidas, 175, 179
Advanced Nanotechnology, 167
aerogels, 63, 64, 107, 111, 112,
    113, 183, 212, 254, 255, 257,
    258
aerosols, 33
Agilent Technologies, 69
Agion Technologies, 61, 62, 104,
    113, 118, 132, 175
AIBO, 140, 141
airbags, 1, 28, 83, 85, 87, 246
aircraft, 246
airline, 246
AK Coatings, 104, 118
Akazawa Japan, 141
Akustica, 41, 135
Akzo Nobel, 115, 122, 257
alcohol, 132
alcohol sensor, 39
Alien Technology, 42
Altair Nanotechnologies, 88
Altria, 246
aluminum oxide, 57
ALZA, 242
AMCOL, 250
American Bowling Service, 195
American Elements, 59

Amorepacific, 158, 159
AMSOIL, 96
analgesic creams, 219
Analog Devices, 27, 28, 29, 137
Andis, 169
Animazoo, 253
anti-aging, 161
anti-bacterial, 60
anti-counterfeit, 252, 255
anti-lock brakes (ABS), 86
anti-microbial, 104, 108, 118,
    132, 176, 219, 240
anti-pollen, 125, 180, 181
anti-rollover systems, 83, 87
Apollo Diamond, 184
Apple, 131, 135, 143
appliances, 59, 62, 104
AppliedSensor, 89
AQUANOVA, 248
Aradigm Corporation, 261
Arc-Com, 115
Architex, 115
Arkema, 49
Armstrong World, 114
Ashland Oil, 90
Asics, 181
Aspen Aerogels, 65, 183
asthma, 217
asthma inhalers, 23, 33
Aston Martin, 94
Astronomy, 190
Asylum Research, 69
Atomic, 68, 209, 263
atomic force microscope (AFM),
    12, 13, 45, 68
atoms, 61
Audi, 89
Audio, 138
Authentix, 256
automotive, 53, 55
Avago Technologies, 42, 129
Avon, 148
avVaa World Health Care
    Products, 166
AXSUN Technologies, 38

Want to Know More?

Listen to the Bourne Report Podcast!

The Bourne Report Podcast discusses real ways that MEMS, nanotechnology and other emerging technologies are changing how we live, work, and play. Listen each week as Marlene Bourne talks about trends relating to the commercial use of MEMS and nanotechnology across all major market segments and industries. New episodes are posted each week.

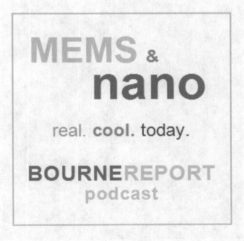

Visit www.bourneresearch.com for more details.

About the Author

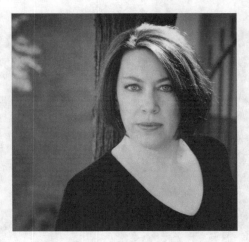

Hollye Schumacher Photography

Marlene Bourne, President & Principal Analyst of Bourne Research is internationally recognized as one of the leading experts on MEMS and its convergence with nanotechnology. With more than a decade of expertise as an industry analyst, her technology and market insight extends from the chip to the end-use product, with both broad and deep knowledge of countless products, companies, markets and applications.

Marlene has provided insight on emerging technologies to many business publications, including *Business 2.0, Business Week, The Economist, Forbes, Investor's Business Daily, Los Angeles Times Magazine, the New York Times* and the *Wall Street Journal*. She has authored numerous articles and is a frequent speaker at conferences and other events.

Marlene holds a Bachelor of Science in Business from the University of Wisconsin—Stout and a Master of Arts in International Business and International Economics from the American University in Washington, DC.

Small is Cool!

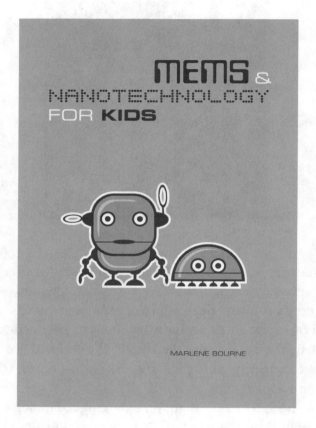

A basic introduction to MEMS and nanotechnology, *MEMS and Nanotechnology for Kids* explores what we can find at the micro- and nano-scale, and then takes a look at various MEMS devices and nanomaterials. Learn how they work and why they're useful in all kinds of products. Written for students age 11-14.

Visit www.bourneresearch.com for more details.

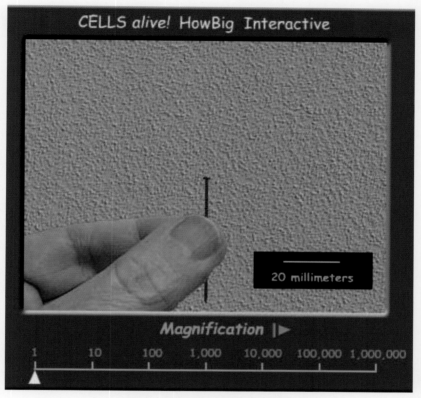

Image courtesy of Quill Graphics

Our journey into the micro- and nano-world begins with a human hand holding a straight pin. The following seven images really put MEMS and nanotechnology into perspective by looking at what we might find on the head of a straight pin (which is about 1–2 millimeters in diameter), by magnifying it one million times its original size.

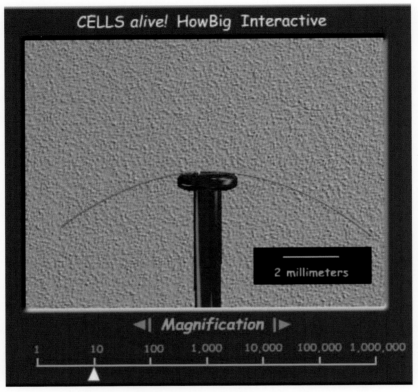

Image courtesy of Quill Graphics

If we magnify the pin by a factor of 10, we not only see a human hair (the diameter of which ranges from 60 to 120 microns), but we can just make out a tiny spec; this is a dust mite, whose width is about 200 microns, also called micrometers.

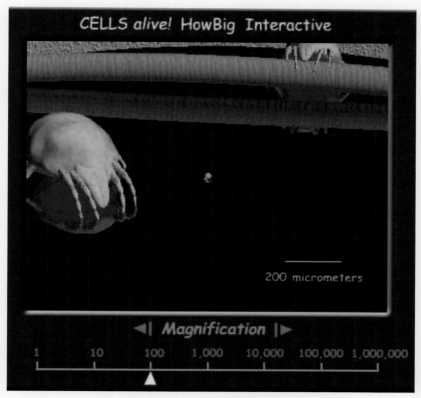

Image courtesy of Quill Graphics

Zooming in by another factor of 10, or now 100 times the original size, the scale of the dust mite and hair is much more apparent. The tiny speck in the middle is a grain of pollen. If you have really good eyesight, you might notice some things next to it.

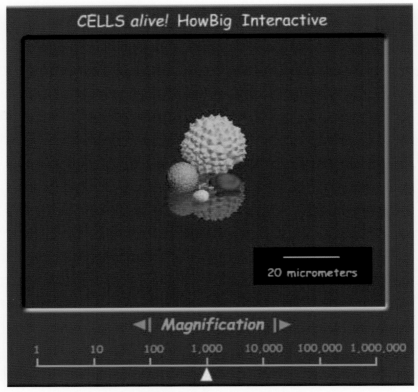

Image courtesy of Quill Graphics

Magnified 1,000 times its original size we now see that the grain of pollen isn't alone on the head of our pin; it towers over a number of other items. The purple ball is a white blood cell, the pink ball is a grain of brewer's yeast and the red disc is a red blood cell. At just 4 micrometers wide, the blood cell, in turn, dwarfs several other really tiny items.

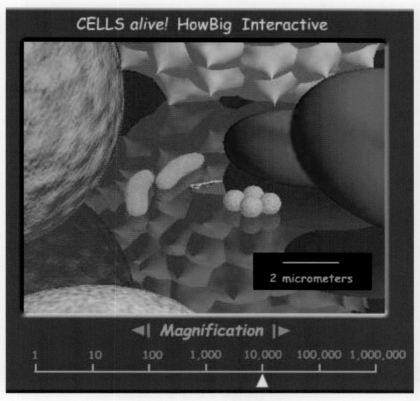

Image courtesy of Quill Graphics

Now that we've zoomed in by a factor of 10,000 we can see what those items next to the red blood cell are. The green caterpillar-like objects are E. coli (bacteria associated with food and waterborne illness) and the 4 yellow balls are staphylococcus (bacteria which causes infections). You might also notice a tiny purple string-like object.

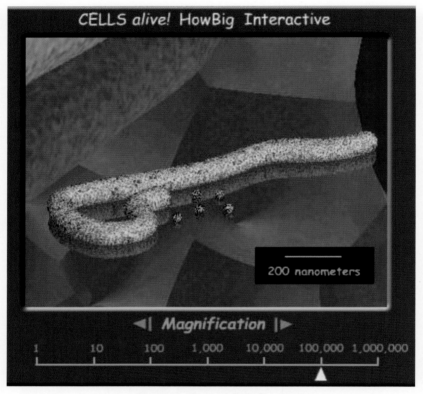

Image courtesy of Quill Graphics

The head of our pin is now magnified 100,000 times its original size. Now we can see that the purple string is in fact a virus—the Ebola virus to be exact. And the four tiny little balls next to it? Those are examples of rhinovirus, the nasty little bug behind the common cold. Let's zoom in one more time.

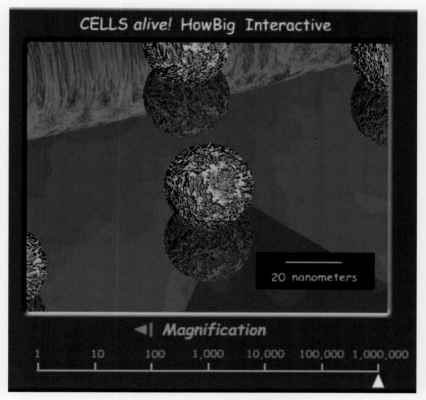

Image courtesy of Quill Graphics

Magnifying our pin one last time, we see how small the cold virus really is: about 20 nanometers in diameter. Keep in mind that the scale of this last image is one million times smaller than the one we started out with. Here is where we could see things like a buckyball or carbon nanotube, both of which are just a few nanometers in diameter.

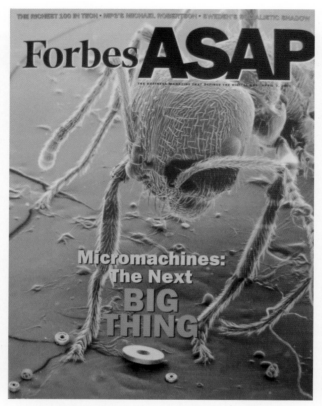

Cover of the April 2, 2001 issue of FORBES ASAP Magazine. The image of an ant towering over several MEMS gears was taken by the late Professor Henry Guckel of the University of Wisconsin—Madison. It provides a great visual scale of how small MEMS devices are.

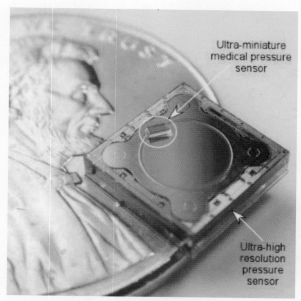

Photo courtesy of Integrated Sensing Systems, Inc.

Small and smaller; two MEMS pressure sensors on a penny.

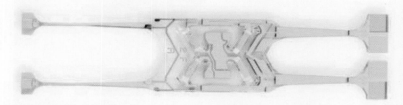

Photo courtesy of Systron Donner Automotive

Close-up of a MEMS gyro sensor. As it senses rotational movement, the two ends almost seem to wiggle slightly up and down, and from side-to-side.

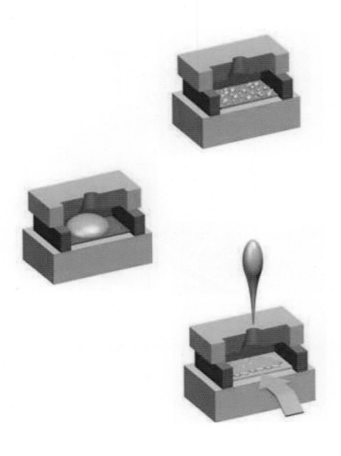

Illustrations courtesy of STMicroelectronics

With thermal ink jet printing technology, ink fills a cavity, which is then heated, creating bubbles (hence the name, thermal bubble). These bubbles of ink are then propelled out of the nozzle onto the paper. The empty cavity fills with ink and the process repeats itself—thousands of times *per second*.

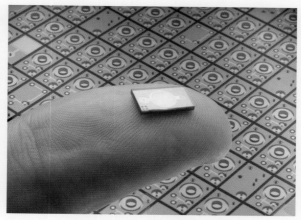

An array of MEMS pumps on a silicon wafer. From Debiotech, the Nanopump™ is inserted just under the skin to deliver insulin, as needed, for up to seven days before being replaced.

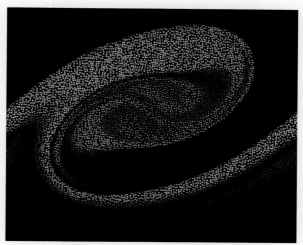

Nanoparticles in Formation[32]

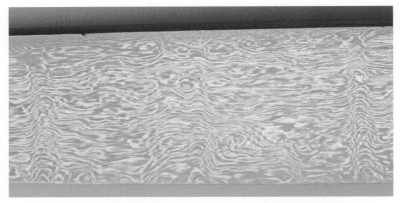

A close-up of the unique pattern of Wootz (Damascus) steel. The design is now known to be the result of carbon nanotubes and other nano-structures[11].

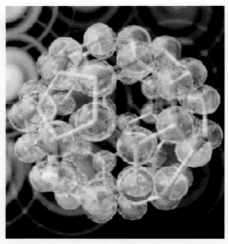

An illustration of a buckyball; notice its soccer ball-like shape?

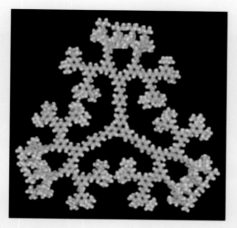

Photo courtesy of Cambridge Display Technology

The snowflake-like shape of a dendrimer.

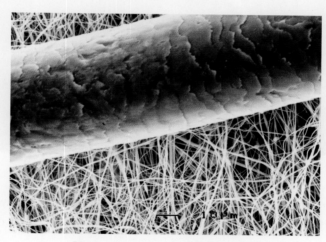

Photo courtesy of eSpin Technologies

Comparing a human hair (in brown) to multiple strands of nanofibers (in white). Keep in mind that human hair has an average diameter of 80 microns.

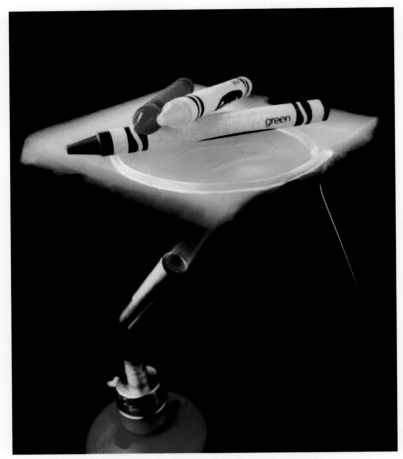

Photo courtesy of NASA Jet Propulsion Laboratory

A sheet of aerogel protects crayons from the heat of a blow torch. Aerogel is naturally a translucent blue—almost the same color as the flame.

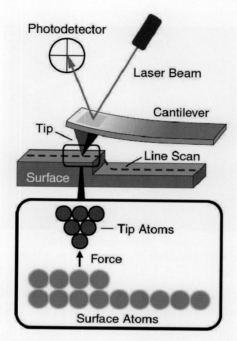

The structure of an atomic force microscope. See how the tip moves along the surface to create an image?

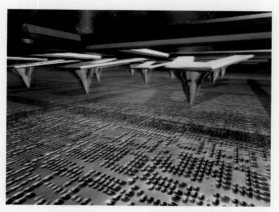

Illustration of IBM's Millipede memory array.

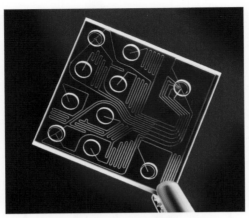

A fairly simple lab-on-a-chip device; liquid samples are injected into the large holes and then move through the micro-channels.

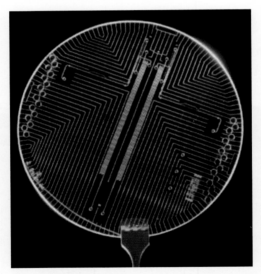

Close-up of a fairly complex lab-on-a-chip device[33].

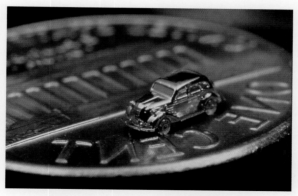

This replica of Toyota's 1936 Model AA Sedan was recognized in 1995 by the Guinness Book of Records as the world's smallest working car. It had 24 individually micromachined parts, including chassis, tires, wheels, axles, headlights, tail lights, bumpers, a spare tire and hubcaps. Its top speed was 10 cm/sec.

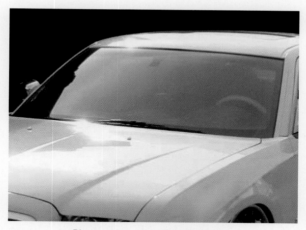

A windshield made of a unique nanocomposite blocks 90 percent of infrared rays and looks cool while you stay cool.

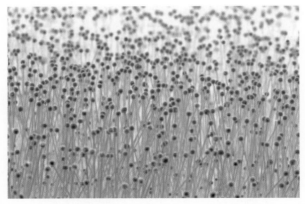

Image courtesy of Oak Ridge National Laboratory (Dr. Zhengwei Pan)

"Nanowire Forest" made from germanium-catalyzed zinc oxide.

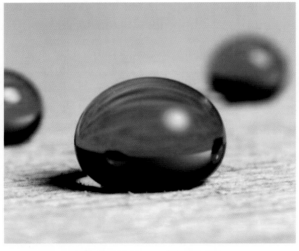

Photo courtesy of BASF AG

The lotus effect means that liquids will remain almost perfectly round on a treated surface, and thus pick up particles of dust and dirt as they roll off that surface.

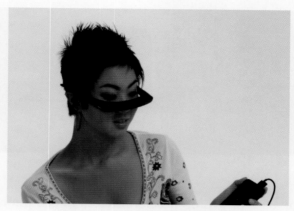

Photo courtesy of myvu Corporation

Watch videos on-the-go with this wearable display from myvu.

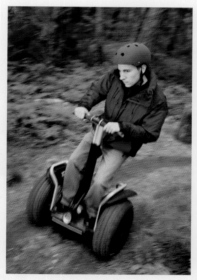

Photo courtesy of Segway LLC

The Segway® Personal Transporter in action. It relies on a combination of MEMS gyro sensors and accelerometers to keep you upright and moving in whatever direction you want to go.

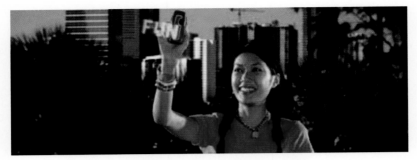

Photo courtesy of Nokia

Two unique uses of MEMS accelerometers in cell phones. In the photo above, you can "air text" simple messages to your friends; type in a short note then wave the phone to project your message. In the photo below, there's no need for a keypad—just "write" the numbers in mid-air. The sensor detects the shape of each number as you move the phone.

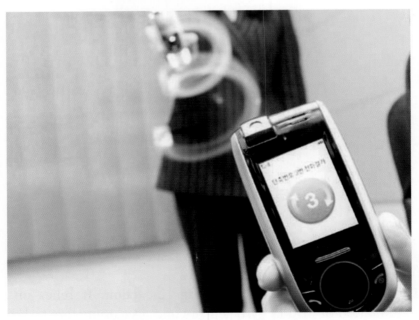

Photo courtesy of Samsung Electronics

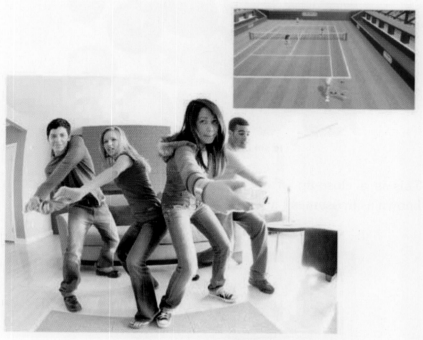

Images courtesy of Nintendo

The Nintendo Wii™ gaming system brings the video gaming experience to a whole new level. Now you can get off the couch and participate in a baseball game, challenge your friends to a lively game of tennis, or even form a bowling league, right in your own living room. A MEMS tri-axis accelerometer (in both the main and secondary remote) is how the Nintendo Wii works its gaming magic.

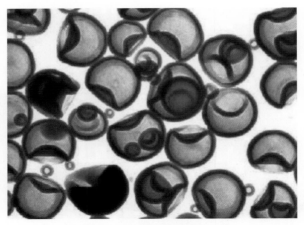

Photo courtesy of NRC Press

This is a close-up of a cluster of vesicles[34] (more commonly known as liposomes); although they're not naturally purple.

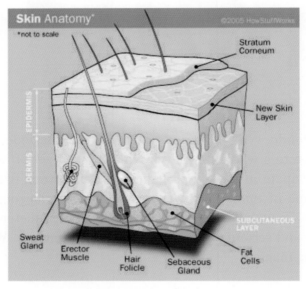

Image courtesy of HowStuffWorks.com

A detailed look at the structure of our skin; most cosmetics can only penetrate the outermost layer.

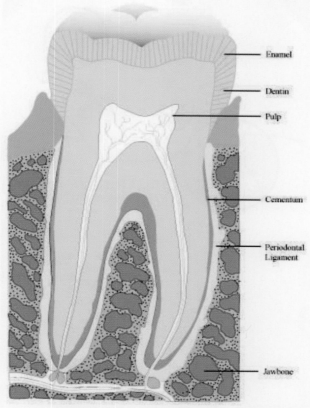

Enamel

Dentin

Pulp

Cementum

Periodontal
Ligament

Jawbone

Image courtesy of National Institute of Dental and Craniofacial Research, National Institutes of Health, Spectrum Series (Biomimetics and Tissue Engineering)

A close-up of the structure of our teeth. Erosion of the cementum (due to receding gums) exposes the main structure of the tooth—the brownish-pink part, called the dentin. This is what causes sensitivity to hot and cold food.

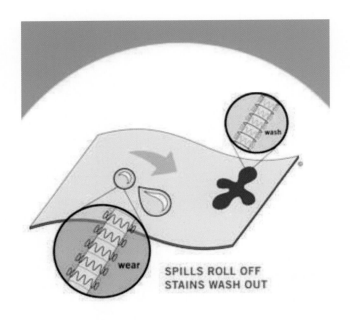

**SPILLS ROLL OFF
STAINS WASH OUT**

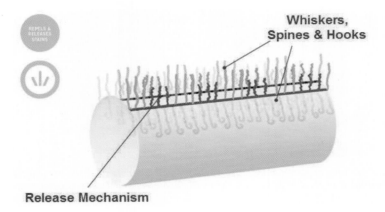

Whiskers,
Spines & Hooks

Release Mechanism

Illustrations courtesy of Nano-Tex, Inc.

The Repels and Releases Stains fabric treatment from Nano-Tex means that liquid spills will bead up and roll off, and any stains you do get (like grass or mud) are easily washed out.

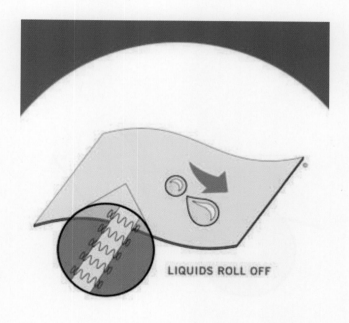

LIQUIDS ROLL OFF

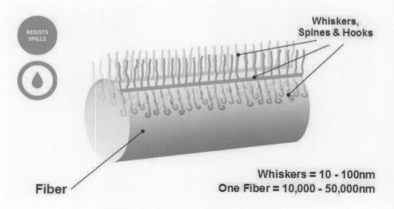

RESISTS
SPILLS

Whiskers,
Spines & Hooks

Fiber

Whiskers = 10 - 100nm
One Fiber = 10,000 - 50,000nm

Illustrations courtesy of Nano-Tex, Inc.

The Resists Spills fabric treatment from Nano-Tex means that liquid spills will bead up and roll off, or can be easily wiped off.

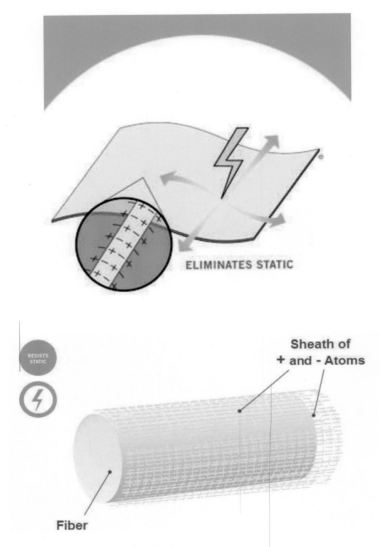

ELIMINATES STATIC

RESISTS STATIC

Sheath of
+ and - Atoms

Fiber

Illustrations courtesy of Nano-Tex, Inc.

The Resists Static fabric treatment eliminates static electricity in synthetic fibers. So, when you pull a fleece cap off your head during the winter, your hair won't stand on end from static.

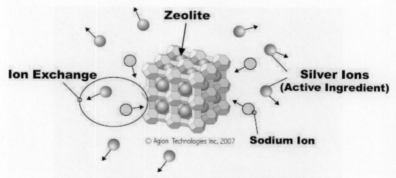

Diagram courtesy of Agion Technologies Inc.

A zeolite is a honeycomb-like structure packed with silver ions. Sodium ions (which are present in moisture) trade spaces with the silver ions, thus releasing the active ingredient necessary to kill most bacteria present.

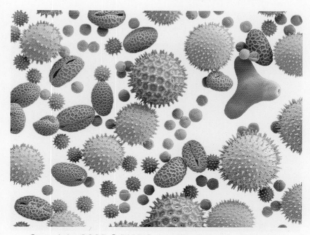

A mixture of pollens. The most common is ragweed, which is the large, prickly-looking yellow ball.

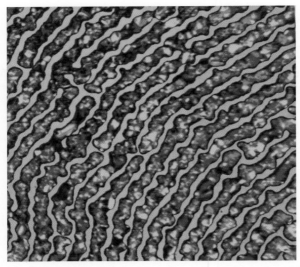

Photo courtesy of Ward Lopes and Heinrich Jaeger, University of Chicago

Self-assembled silver nanowires.

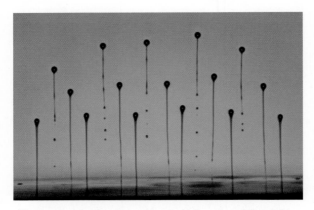

Photo taken by Dr. Steve Hoath, University of Cambridge

A close-up view of ink being propelled out of the nozzles of an ink jet cartridge. This photo was part of the Epson Photography Competition at the University of Cambridge.

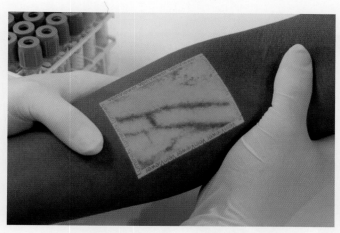

The use of Texas Instruments' DLP®, in combination with infrared light, illuminates the veins present just below the skin so technicians can insert needles or catheters more precisely.

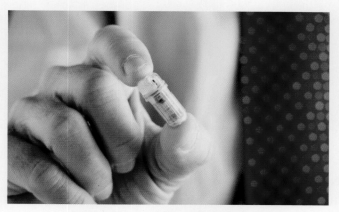

Photo courtesy of SmartPill Corporation

Doctors can now obtain detailed images of the gastrointestinal tract with the use of the SmartPill, which patients swallow. The pill transmits data as it works its way through the intestines.

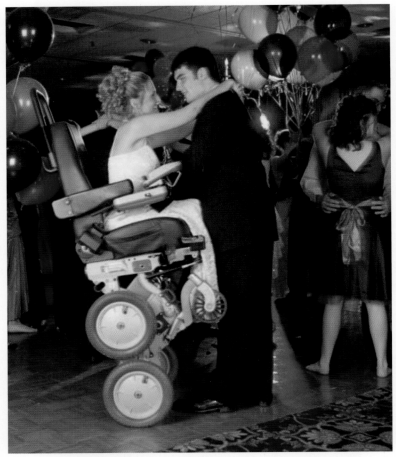

Photo courtesy of Independence Technology LLC

The INDEPENDENCE® iBOT® Mobility System, one of the most unique wheelchairs ever developed, relies on multiple MEMS gyro sensors and accelerometers to provide balance. Because of this, the chair is able to lift its user to a standing height and balance on just two wheels. This allows the person in the wheelchair to do things we might take for granted, such as dancing at a high-school prom.

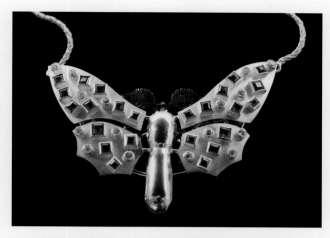

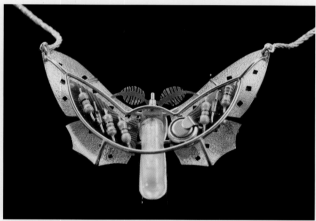

Photos courtesy of Sensory Design and Technology Ltd.

This unique pendant automatically provides a mist of perfume. It
works via the use of a tiny lab-on-a-chip device and a MEMS
humidity sensor.

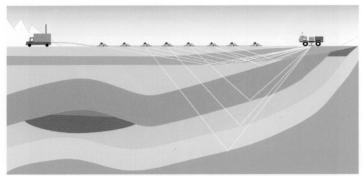

Illustration courtesy of Sercel

MEMS geophones (placed at even intervals) create a map of various underground layers so geologists can find pockets of oil.

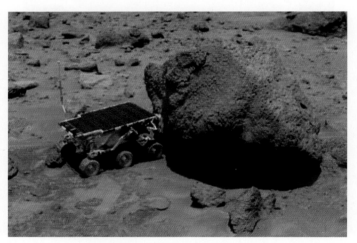

Photo courtesy of NASA/JPL-Caltech

In July 1997, during the Mars Pathfinder mission, the rover Sojourner examined a rock called Yogi. MEMS gyro sensors helped this unique explorer navigate on the red planet.